Corneal Transplantation

Corneal Transplantation

Frank M. Polack, M.D., F.A.C.S.

Professor of Ophthalmology
Department of Ophthalmology
College of Medicine
University of Florida
Gainesville, Florida

and

Consultant in Ophthalmology
Veterans Administration Hospital
Gainesville, Florida

and

Medical Director
North Florida Lions Eye Bank
Gainesville, Florida

GRUNE & STRATTON

A Subsidiary of Harcourt Brace Jovanovich, Publishers
New York □ San Francisco □ London

Corneal Transplantation

Frank M. Polack, M.D., F.A.C.S.

Professor of Ophthalmology
Department of Ophthalmology
College of Medicine
University of Florida
Gainesville, Florida

and

Consultant in Ophthalmology
Veterans Administration Hospital
Gainesville, Florida

and

Medical Director
North Florida Lions Eye Bank
Gainesville, Florida

GRUNE & STRATTON

A Subsidiary of Harcourt Brace Jovanovich, Publishers
New York □ San Francisco □ London

Library of Congress Cataloging in Publication Data

Polack, Frank M   1929-
  Corneal transplantation.

  Bibliography: p.
  Includes index.
  1. Cornea—Transplantation.   I. Title. [DNLM:
1. Cornea—Transplantation.   WW220 P762c]
RE80.P64   617.7'19   77-15622
ISBN 0-8089-1048-5

Grune & Stratton, Inc.
111 Fifth Avenue
New York, New York 10003

Distributed in the United Kingdom by
Academic Press, Inc. (London) Ltd.
24/28 Oval Road, London NW1

Library of Congress Catalog Number 77-15622
International Standard Book Number 0-8089-1048-5

Printed in the United States of America

To my wife Patricia, and to my sons
Frank Edward, Peter Joseph, and William
Anthony

Corneal transplantation, when performed in favorable host tissue, accounts for the most successful type of organ transplantation. Possibly over 3000 keratoplasties are done annually in the United States, and it is evident that the number of potential recipients is on the increase. Surgeons subspecialized in areas of surgery should become true experts in their fields, and this must include a full knowledge of all basic and experimental information. Training fellowships, therefore, should not stress surgical expertise alone, but academic competence as well. Surgeons being trained as corneal specialists should acquire adequate background in the field of corneal transplantation in order to obtain the best clinical results. This book is aimed toward the developing corneal surgeon as well as the corneal investigator, and it contains basic and practical clinical information. It presents an overview of several parameters that influence the acceptance of corneal grafts and the mechanisms by which they fail to remain clear.

The text is divided into four parts: Part I deals with the basic problems in tissue transplantation and the biology of the corneal graft; Part 2 is concerned with techniques and instrumentation; Part 3 discusses the influence of host response in clinical results and the pathology of the graft; and Part 4 presents information pertaining to the donor tissue, its preservation, and how to organize and operate an eye bank. Studies on the fate of corneal grafts, done several years ago in collaboration with Dr. George K. Smelser, and described in Part I, are still pertinent. This section on the biology of the corneal graft has been updated by the inclusion of newer immunological concepts. In these and in the chapters on microsurgical techniques and the pathology of failed grafts, I try to point out the need to develop the concept of keratoplasty as a truly microsurgical operative procedure. This is borne of many years of personal experimental work, teaching microsurgical techniques and my clinical experience at the University of Florida for the past ten years.

Foreword

In the past 10 to 20 years there has been a marked increase in the percentage of successful corneal transplants in man. This has resulted from our increased knowledge of the physiology of the normal cornea, the causes of early and late graft failure, improved donor material, and better surgical techniques and instrumentation. Much of this expanded knowledge has resulted from the excellent experimental studies in animals and clinical observations in man by Dr. Frank Polack. His reports and those of others which have accounted for these advances are published in numerous ophthalmic and other medical journals. Thus, the student with a beginning interest in corneal grafting, or the experienced surgeon who wishes to keep abreast of modern advances, must refer to multiple journals to accomplish these aims. This book by Dr. Polack is therefore very timely.

The Table of Contents clearly describes the material in this publication, but beyond that it should be pointed out that Dr. Polack has included a superb review of the literature on each of these subjects and has added his first-hand knowledge, which resulted from his own experimentation, to many of the scientific advances. A few of the latter are regeneration of the cornea after injury, the mechanisms involved in the allograft rejection, techniques for corneal transplantation, and the selection and preservation of donor corneal material.

This is an important publication not only for the ophthalmic surgeon interested in corneal transplantation, but also for those persons who will be involved in the referral and postoperative care of individuals who need corneal grafting.

A. E. Maumenee, M.D.

Acknowledgments

In addition to Dr. George K. Smelser, who introduced me to the field of experimental pathology of the eye (see the studies described in Part 1), I had the invaluable assistance of the following colleagues from Columbia University: Drs. V. Manski, H. Cardona, L. Khorazo, Ms. J. Rose and Miss V. Ozanics. My deep appreciation is also extended to Dr. A. G. DeVoe and Dr. Ramon Castroviejo, to whom I owe my early clinical experience in clinical corneal pathology. The enthusiasm of Dr. Castroviejo originated more than one research project in this area.

The histopathology of the corneal graft could not have been presented here without the invaluable collaboration of Dr. H. Inomata and Dr. A. Kanai, who performed the transmission electron microscopic studies. My thanks are also extended to Drs. H. E. Kaufman, W. Townsend, J. McEntyre, F. Brightbill, S. Waltman, R. Abel, P. Binder, Ch. Wind, C. West, H. Hawa, R. Vidal, R. Charlin, C. Siverio, J. Sanchez, Y. Centifanto, and others who have contributed or collaborated with me in some projects. Dr. Donald Willard merits my special thanks because he stimulated the publication of this book and made valuable critical comments on the manuscript.

The tremendous task of transcribing and editing the manuscript for over a year was done almost exclusively by Mrs. Patty DeYot. Mrs. Eileen Giffin did the final transcription of the text. Bibliographical research and editing was done by Miss Suzanne Heard, and technical photographic work by Mrs. Maruja McNiece. Miss Roxann Crocco edited the chapter on the organization of the Eye Bank. My thanks to these collaborators.

Appreciation is also extended to the staff of Grune & Stratton for their excellent cooperation and efficient and fast work that made the production of this book a pleasant event.

Dr. A. E. Maumenee opened the doors to the study of corneal transplantation and immune reaction. I am very honored by his acceptance to write the Foreword.

Contents

Introduction

The replacement of totally opaque corneas due to disease or trauma by clear animal corneas was the dream of eye physicians for several centuries. Their endeavors were then limited by medical, ethical, religious, and technical barriers. Transplantation of corneal tissue began in 1837 when Bigger[1] attempted this procedure in animals, but the first human graft wasn't performed until 1872 when Power[2] performed the operation in England, followed by others in Europe and Russia in the late 19th and early 20th centuries. Further advances in keratoplasty were mostly due to improvements in instrumentation and surgical techniques, and many surgeons[3-7] proved the feasibility of corneal homo-transplantation; however, the incidence of postoperative complications leading to cloudiness of the graft were still high.

Basic questions pertinent to the biology of the corneal graft were raised in the early 1940s and were amply discussed by Paufique and collaborators in a classical monograph.[8] Obtaining a clear graft without complications at that time was a triumph, since early clouding of the graft occurred frequently. This problem attracted the attention of many surgeons when opacification occurred without obvious reasons two or more weeks after transplantation. It was for this group of grafts that the term "maladie du Greffon" was applied following the description of Paufique et al. It was about this time that Medawar[9] demonstrated that the rejection of skin grafts was due to an immunologic process and that this phenomenon would also apply to other tissue grafts. This information was applied to the problem of corneal grafting by Maumenee[10] and Mueller and Maumenee[11] who opened the door for the study of mechanisms of corneal graft rejection and other causes of opacification, such as donor tissue viability.

The information obtained in recent years from clinical and experimental investigation, and the application of microsurgical techniques, have made corneal transplantation a reliable procedure with predictable results. A corneal surgeon today must give attention not only to the surgical techniques, but also to the type and quality of instruments and sutures and, principally, to the biologic and immunologic factors that influence graft survival.

Although the concepts of graft success were different in 1960, the studies that form the basis of this book began at that time. We believed then that the main cause of graft opacification was the immune reaction, and this is true today. However, at that time, many nonimmunologic causes of graft failure were labeled as graft rejection. It was important then to investigate the reasons why grafts failed. Parallel to this was the need to learn why corneal grafts could succeed and what was necessary to obtain optically useful grafts.

Animal experimentation is the key to recognizing and improving technical problems in corneal transplantation, but it is also the basis for understanding the biologic problems pertinent to wound healing, tissue repair, and the immune reaction. Therefore, it seems valid to use experimental evidence to establish some principles that must be followed in keratoplasty and, possibly, in any type of corneal surgery. Surgery modifies the biology and physiology of the tissue involved. In corneal transplantation, we are working at the cellular level, and we must use the least traumatic surgical technique and the best instruments to realize our purpose with minimal cell or tissue destruction. The same applies to obtaining donor tissue, preparing the host, et cetera.

The purpose of this book, therefore, is to present the reader with a sequential study of the many factors to be considered for a successful keratoplasty in the human.

REFERENCES

1. Bigger SLL: An inquiry into the possibility of transplanting the cornea, with the view of relieving blindness (hitherto deemed incurable) caused by several diseases of that structure. Dublin J Med Sci 11:408, 1837

2. Power H: On transplantation of the cornea. Rep Internat Ophth Cong, 1972, London, 4, 1873, pp. 172-176

3. Paton RT: Keratoplasty. New York, McGraw-Hill, 1955

4. Trevor-Roper PD: "The History of Corneal Grafting." In Casey TA (ed): Corneal Grafting. London, Butterworths, 1972, p. 1-10

5. Dhanda RP, Kalevar, V (eds): In Corneal Surgery. International Ophthalmology Clinics. Boston, Little, Brown, 1972

6. Offret F, Pouliquen Y: Les Homogreffes de la Cornee. Paris, Masson et Cie, 1974

7. Puchovskaya N: Corneal Transplantation in Complicated Leukomas. Moscow, Peace, 1969

8. Paufique L, Sourdille GP, Offret G: Les Greffes de la Cornee. Paris, Masson et Cie, 1948

9. Medawar P: Immunity to homologous grafted skin III: The fate of skin homografts transplanted to the brain, to subcutaneous tissue, and to the anterior chamber of the eye. Br J Exp Pathol 29:58, 1948

10. Maumenee AE: Influence of donor-recipient sensitization on corneal grafts. Am J Ophthalmol 34:142, 1951

11. Mueller H, Maumenee AE: Considerations sur la maladie du Greffon. Arch Ophthalmol (Paris) 11:146, 1951

PART 1

Basic Problems in Tissue Transplantation and the Biology of the Corneal Graft

Chapter 1

Experimental Corneal Grafts

Experimental keratoplasty in laboratory animals presents many problems that are not found in humans and that tend to discourage the surgeon working in this field for the first time. Fixation of grafts was one of the main problems in the past, but today, with the use of the operating microscope and finer suture material, consistently good results can be obtained. The anesthesia of the animal is perhaps the most common problem, followed by infections or dislocations of the graft. Even though experiments are frequently done in corneal grafts, a review of the literature reveals few papers describing experimental keratoplasties,[1-10] one of the most extensive studies being that of Castroviejo in 1937.[4]

Keratoplasty in the experimental animal is a required exercise in understanding the technical problems of this type of surgery, particularly when working under the operating microscope. Experimental keratoplasty is not only useful as surgical training, but is also a means for studying the biology of the corneal graft.

The surgical techniques for experimental keratoplasties in the rabbit are well known in many medical centers dedicated to the investigation of immunologic problems in corneal transplantation. With few exceptions, the operation is essentially similar to that performed in the human. In our laboratory, we use edge-to-edge sutures to fix the graft; however, in previous years, we have used appositional sutures, which also give good results, particularly in rats and guinea pigs. The two techniques will be described below.

MATERIALS AND METHODS

The Experimental Animal

Rabbits are the most frequently used animals because of their availability, easy handling, and the size of their eyes. It is convenient to use adult rabbits (4–5-mo-old) because their eyes will have attained good size, and they will be more resistant to anesthesia. If albino rabbits are used, they should weigh about 3–4 kg, the fur should be clean and smooth, and their ears free of mites. Animals should be kept in large wire cages with abundant food and water. Dehydration is a frequent cause of death, particularly after anesthesia. Animal handlers should be informed about the surgical procedure to be done, so the rabbits can be carefully moved when the cage is being cleaned. Failure to do this will cause dislocated and infected grafts.

Similar care and precaution must be followed with larger animals. Some procedures, the size of the cages, and lodging of experimental animals must follow the regulations promulgated by the Department of Health, Education and Welfare Public Health Service.

Instruments

1 Eyelid retractor (small wire speculum)
2 Mosquito clamps
2 Fixation forceps (0.9 teeth) or Bishop-Harmon (1 × 1)
1 Trephine blade (6 or 7 mm)
1 Corneal scissors (Castroviejo—single curve; Storz E3220, Weck 2-270, Sparta 12-382)
1 Suture scissors
1 Forceps, corneal (0.12 mm teeth)
1 Needle holder (standard for 4'0' silk)
1 Needle holder (Microsurgical)
1 Saline solution irrigator (or one 10cc syringe)
1 Tuberculin syringe (for heparin drip)
   Sutures (4'0', 8'0', or 10'0')

Drugs and Medications

Recommended drugs and medications are atropine 1%, Neo-synephrine 10%, sodium pentothal (30 mg/kg), heparin (10,000 U/cu cm), Neosporin® solution, normal saline solution, and Chlorpromazine (Thorazine).

Anesthesia

Rabbits (3 kg) are premedicated with 10 mg/kg of Thorazine i.m. 1 hr before surgery. Twenty minutes before surgery, the pupils are dilated with 10% Neo-synephrine and 1% atropine. The animals are then anesthetized with intravenous sodium pentothal (30 mg/kg). The anesthetic is injected slowly into the lateral vein of the ear using a 27-G butterfly needle with a polyethylene tube adapter (Fig. 1-1). This needle can remain in place after being secured with adhesive tape to allow the surgeon to continue the injection of the anesthetic if it is required. The injection of the anesthetic is stopped as soon as the rabbit's ears drop. The animal should not jump when the ear is pinched. Intravenous anesthesia can be supplemented with ether if necessary. A plastic cup with perforations at the bottom and half filled with cotton is an effective ether mask. Others prefer the use of cyclopropane anesthesia solely through a funnel-like mask. Once the rabbit has been anesthetized, the hairs around the eye and the eyelashes are trimmed and flushed away with water. The conjunctiva is rinsed with saline solution.

Sterile technique should follow, but in my experience, gloves and mask are not necessary for the surgeon. Drapes over the animal are advisable, but infections do not seem to increase by not using them.

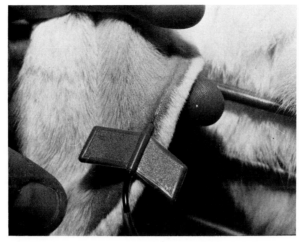

Figure 1-1.   Butterfly needle (27-G) used to inject pentosol in the marginal ear vein of the rabbit.

OPERATIVE TECHNIQUES

Keratoplasty With Continuous and Interrupted Sutures

Surgery is started when the pupil is fully dilated and after the application of several drops of an antibiotic solution. The animal is positioned under the operating microscope and the lids retracted with 4′0′ silk sutures or a wire speculum. Two 4′0′ silk sutures are passed through the superior and inferior rectus muscles and secured to the drapes with small mosquito clamps. The most convenient graft sizes for experimental studies are 6½ and 7 mm. Grafts larger than 8 mm have a higher tendency to peripheral synechiae. Trephination of the cornea is best done with an assistant holding the globe with a fixation forceps at the insertion of the inferior rectus suture, while the surgeon holds the eye at the 12-o'clock position, thus preventing the eye from rotating and producing an imperfect cut (Fig. 1-2). Due to the steepness of the rabbit cornea, the depth gauge of the trephine is useless; therefore, it is necessary to use a trephine without plunger. One must trephine carefully and watch for and stop at the first gush of fluid around the blade, which indicates a partial penetration into the anterior chamber. One or two drops of heparin (10,000 U/cc) or fresh 1% sodium citrate injected into the anterior chamber is enough to prevent clotting of aqueous fluid for 10–20 min (Fig. 1-3). Removal of the corneal button is completed with the corneal scissors (Fig. 1-4). The donor tissue can be obtained from another rabbit eye in the same manner if two simultaneous grafts are done, or after excising the cornea from an enucleated eye by cutting the graft endothelial side up with a corneal punch (see chapter 8). Interrupted or continuous sutures with 8′0′ silk material or 10′0′ monofilament nylon are used (Fig. 1-5); however, silk must be removed in 7–10 days, otherwise severe vascularization will occur. Usually, the anterior chamber does not require saline injection except when it

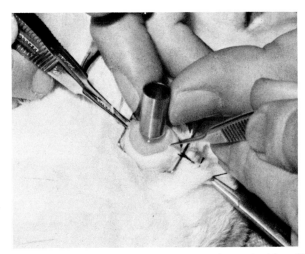

Figure 1-2. Corneal trephination is performed with a disposable blade. The cut can be observed through the microscope. An assistant helps to steady the eye.

appears to be very shallow at the end of the procedure. Postoperatively, the eye is treated with atropine ointment and a topical antibiotic for 3–4 days. Nylon sutures can be left in place for 10–14 days.

Keratoplasty With Splint (Appositional) Sutures

The eye is fixed with two 4'0' silk sutures at 12- and 6-o'clock. A superficial cut is made on the corneal epithelium with the trephine, in order to use this circle as a guide for the double cross sutures that will retain the graft. The

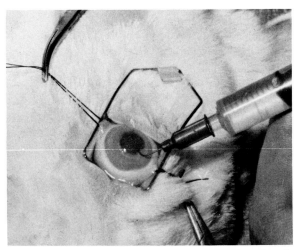

Figure 1-3. A partial penetration of the anterior chamber, enough to introduce corneal scissors, has been obtained with the trephine. A few drops of heparin are injected into the anterior chamber to avoid aqueous humor clotting.

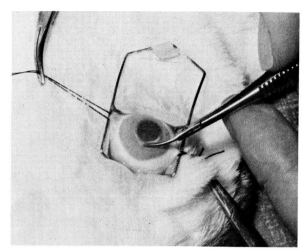

Figure 1-4. The corneal button is excised with single-curve Castroviejo corneal scissors.

sutures should lie just inside the graft edge and its exact location indicated by markings of a caliper placed near the limbus (Fig. 1-6**A**). The two sets of sutures (Davis & Geck, CE-2 6′0′ silk) must cross through a thin polyethylene film (Fig. 1-6**B**) so they will not rest over the graft. Once the preplaced sutures are completed, they are pulled to one side, and the cornea is trephined in the previously marked area (Fig. 1-6**C**). There is no need for anticoagulant solution if the donor graft is already cut; but if a delay of a few minutes is expected, it will be necessary to instill a few drops of recently prepared sterile 1% sodium citrate in the anterior chamber. A clot will form shortly after the graft is in place, and the two sutures are tied, thereby securing the graft. Additional locking sutures must be placed at each corner of the square splint suture (Fig. 1-6**D**). Eyes are cleaned

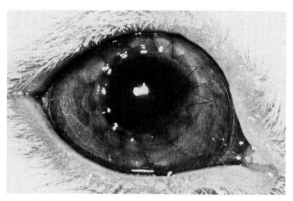

Figure 1-5. Corneal graft sutured with 10′0′ monofilament nylon in a running fashion. The silk sutures have been removed.

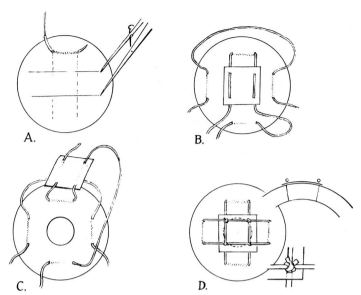

Figure 1-6. The technique of penetrating keratoplasty fixed by means of a double set of crossed sutures and a polyethylene film splint. The width of the set of double sutures should be 0.5 mm smaller than the diameter of the graft. Davis & Geck 6′0′ silk sutures with a long reverse cutting needle were used in this experiment. The diagram shows how the polyethylene film is secured with one set of sutures. These are pulled apart for trephination of the cornea, and immediately after the graft is in place, the sutures and the splint are secured in place. Locking sutures are placed at the intersection of the main sutures over the polyethylene film as shown in **B**.

daily followed by the instillation of an antibiotic solution. The sutures and the splint are removed 6–7 days later (Fig. 1-7). Figure 1-8 shows the instruments used.

COMMENT

In 1963, I reported the results of several means of fixating corneal grafts using various types of sutures available at that time, as well as various suturing techniques that had been used in humans.[7] Some of them (splint sutures) had already been discarded with the development of new corneal needles in the early 1950s. However, it was the purpose of the experiments to find a way to fixate the grafts with the least amount of trauma to its stromal and endothelial borders so we could determine the number of cells surviving keratoplasty. Edge-to-edge or running sutures (7′0′ silk) destroyed too many donor cells to be used in these experiments. Graft fixation with large contact lenses sutured to the host, even though feasible, induced a high rate of infection. Our best results were obtained by fixating the graft with preplaced sutures from limbus to limbus over a protective polyethylene film. Since this suture was preplaced, fixation of the graft was very rapid with a minimum of tissue manipulation and instantaneous restoration of the anterior chamber. A similar method had been used by Filatov,[11] Stallard,[12] Sourdille,[13] and Dolhman[15] to fixate the graft, and a method using an egg mem-

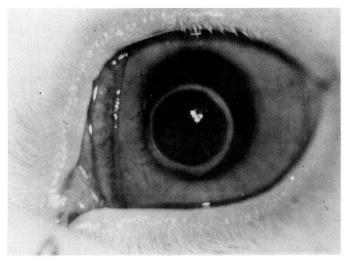

Figure 1-7. Clear penetrating graft (5.5 mm) in an albino rabbit 4 wk after keratoplasty.

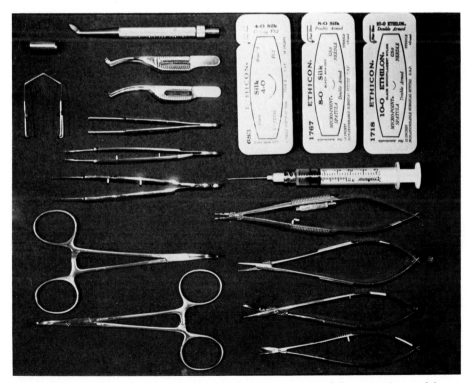

Figure 1-8. Microsurgical instruments and sutures required for experimental kerato-plasty.

brane placed under the sutures had been implemented by Thomas,[2] Castroviejo,[3] and others. I found this technique useful to fixate small grafts in rats or guinea pigs. In the rabbit, the ideal method today is that of interrupted or continuous sutures as described.

The percentage of clear grafts obtained with the splint-fixation method in rabbits was approximately 60% with grafts over 6 mm and 75% with grafts of smaller size. This was the technique employed in over 200 experimental grafts for the purpose of studying the persistency of their cellular components.[11] Since then, finer suture material, such as 8'0' and 9'0' silk and 9'0' and 10'0' monofilament nylon, have become available with spatulated needles, and reports of experimental corneal grafting in rabbits,[8] dogs,[9] and monkeys[10] have been published. With the newer needles and sutures, microsurgical instruments and the operating microscope, it is now possible to do large grafts in rabbits or smaller animals with edge-to-edge sutures and obtain excellent results.

Types of Corneal Grafts

Penetrating or full-thickness grafts have been used in these studies; however, there are other types of corneal transplants (Fig. 1-9), called *lamellar* or partial thickness, when several lamellae of the cornea are replaced. If grafts replace only a portion of the cornea, they are called partial grafts. Usually they vary in size from 7 to 9 mm in diameter, the most common sizes used clinically being 7.5 mm and 8.0 mm. These partial transplants may be central or eccentric.

Partially penetrating or lamellar transplants may serve a tectonic, rather than optical, purpose. They are used to reinforce diseased or very thin corneal tissue, such as advanced keratoconus or extensive ulceration, and are usually done in preparation for penetrating keratoplasties. These transplants could have

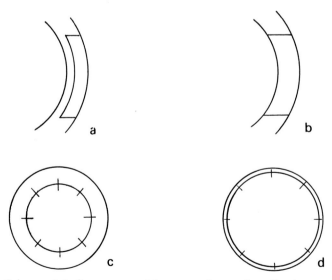

Figure 1-9. Schema **A** indicates a partial penetrating or lamellar keratoplasty; in **B** a fully penetrating or full-thickness keratoplasty; **C** shows a partial keratoplasty; **D** total keratoplasty.

optical purposes when they replace excised portions of opaque host cornea. The thickness of the donor tissue may vary from 0.3 to 0.4 mm, but sometimes the "lamellar" donor is a full-thickness graft without the endothelium. The donor lamellar graft does not have to be viable. At the present time, most surgeons use "outdated" (over 5 days old) refrigerated corneal tissue, glycerol-preserved corneas, or frozen (−79°C or −110°C) corneas without preserving solutions (see chapter 16).

As a rule, penetrating keratoplasties are smaller than the diameter of the cornea, because total corneal replacement has a much higher incidence of rejection.

There are also atypical corneal transplants for certain pathologic conditions, such as peripheral corneal degenerations or marginal ulcers. These transplants may have a half-moon or C shape, be donut-shaped, oval, etc.

REFERENCES

1. Leoz-Ortin G: Algunos estudios y ensayos sobre queratoplastias. Acta IX Asamblea Soc Hisp Am 18:161, 1914
2. Thomas WT: Transplantation of the cornea: A preliminary report on a series of experiments on rabbits, together with a demonstration of four rabbits with clear corneal grafts. Trans Ophthalmol Soc UK 50:127, 1930
3. Castroviejo R: Estudio experimental en conejos con corneas leucomatosas. Trans Int Congr Ophthalmol (Madrid) 1:78, 1933
4. Castroviejo R: Keratoplasty. Microscopic study of the corneal grafts. Trans Am Ophthalmol Soc 35:355, 1937
5. Stansbury F, Wadsworth JA: Corneal transplantation in rabbits. Am J Ophthalmol 30:968, 1947
6. Greaves DP: Experimental penetrating keratoplasty. Collt Repr Inst Ophthalmol, London 7, 1954–1955, p 135
7. Polack FM: Queratoplastia experimental. Arch Soc Oftal Hisp Amer (Spain) 23:758, 1963
8. Khodadoust AA: Penetrating keratoplasty in the rabbit. Am J Ophthalmol 66:899, 1968
9. McEntyre JM: Experimental penetrating keratoplasty in the dog. Arch Ophthalmol 8:372–376, 1968
10. Sanchez J, Polack FM, Eve R, et al: Corneal endothelial healing and posterior wound closure after "through and through" suturing. Can J Ophthalmol 9:48, 1974
11. Filatov VP: Transplantation of the cornea. Arch Ophthalmol 13:321, 1935
12. Stallard HB: Eye Surgery. Baltimore, Williams & Wilkins, 1958
13. Sourdille GP, Paufique L, Offret G: Les Greffes de la Cornee. Paris, Masson et Cie, 1948, p 144
14. Polack FM, Smelser GK, Rose J: Long term survival of isotopically labeled stromal and endothelial cells in corneal homografts. Am J Ophthalmol 57:67, 1964
15. Dohlman CH: On the fate of the corneal graft. Acta Ophthalmol 35:286, 1957

Chapter 2

The Fate of Transplanted Corneal Tissue

ANATOMICAL CONSIDERATIONS

We can assume that the reader is familiar with the structure of the cornea; however, a brief review of its anatomy seems pertinent here because we will study not only the survival of the various components of the corneal graft, but also mechanisms of wound healing and pathologic changes in failed grafts.

Epithelium

Ultramicroscopic studies of corneal epithelium suggest that the surface structure is intimately related to the presence of a normal tear film layer. The surface corneal epithelium is covered by minute folds that may aid in holding the tear film. In the dry eye, these folds disappear. The cytoplasm of these cells have fibrils. An increase in the number of fibrils is seen in cells producing keratin. This anomaly is seen in vitamin-A deficient eyes. The deepest epithelial cells are engaged in protein synthesis. Cells attach one another by their interdigitation and by desmosomes (tonofibrils), and rest on a basement membrane (BM) 300–600 Å thick to which they attach by small fibrils called hemidesmosomes (Fig. 2-1). This layer is manufactured by the epithelial cell, it is composd of collagenous material and glycoprotein, and it is one of the most important elements in maintaining the integrity of the epithelial layer. Lack of BM synthesis or its deposition over an abnormal surface (scar tissue) causes recurrent detachment of the epithelium. The turnover of epithelial cells in primates is around 10 days and between 7 and 10 days in rabbits.

Bowman's Layer

In the human eye this layer measures 10–14 μ. It is a portion of differentiated stroma composed of fine collagen fibrils, compacted within proteoglycan substance. Its anterior surface is covered by the basement membrane of the epithelium, and its internal surface merges with the fibers of the corneal stroma (Fig. 2-1).

Stroma

The collagen that forms the stroma of the cornea is arranged in parallel fibrils, these in turn arrange themselves in bundles and form lamellae (Fig. 2-2). Collagen bundles criss-cross in various directions from limbus to limbus while

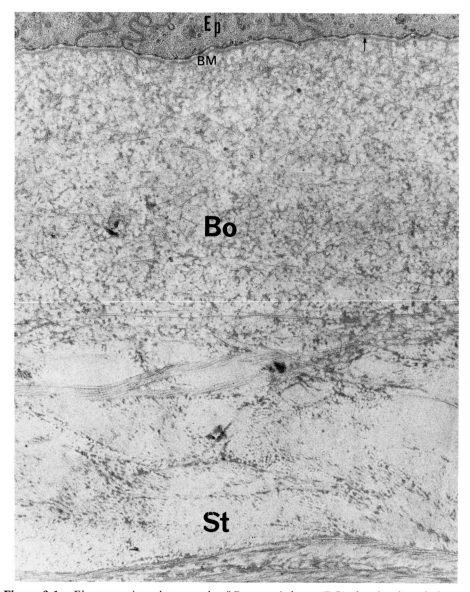

Figure 2-1. Electron microphotograph of Bowman's layer (BO) showing its relation to the epithelium basement membrane (BM) and superficial stroma (ST) of rhesus monkey cornea. The epithelium is attached to the BM by hemidesmosomes (arrow). (× 15,000; courtesy of Dr. A. Kanai)

moving from one layer to another, as in the weave of a basket (Fig. 2-3). Cleavage planes are easily found for lamellar dissections. They are easier to dissect towards the posterior layer of the cornea. Near the limbus, some collagen bundles are arranged circularly (1.5 mm). These bundles do not stretch in keratoconus as do radial fibers. The basic collagen unit is called tropocollagen; it consists of three strands of equal length, each containing about 1000 amino acids. They are

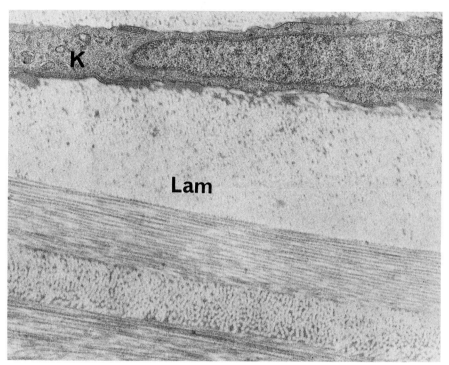

Figure 2-2. Stroma of rhesus monkey cornea showing a keratocyte (K) within collagen fibrils that form a bundle or a lamellae (LAM). Fibrils change in orientation in alternate lamellae. The surgical lamellae (macroscopic) are composed of several of these fine bundles (×20,000; courtesy of Dr. A. Kanai).

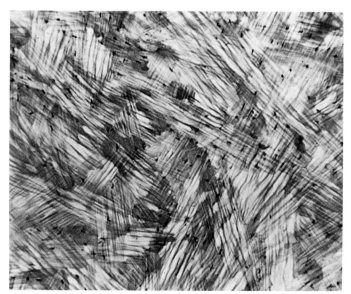

Figure 2-3. Tangential section of central area of rabbit cornea showing collagen bundles criss-crossing at various angles. This is the appearance of a thin (8–10 μ) lamellae (silver carbonate of del Rio Hortega, ×100).

called alpha chains, each one being made of ⅓ glycine, ⅓ proline and hydroxyproline, and ⅓ other amino acids (Fig. 4-23). In our studies of collagen survival and turnover, we used radioactive glycine (^{14}C) to label these elementary collagen components. Variations in the amino acid's arrangement in each chain makes the type of collagen that is characteristic of embryonic tissue, cornea, skin, etc. In the chapter on wound healing we have summarized the biochemical steps for the synthesis of collagen. The corneal collagen is quite characteristic due to its uniform diameter (340 Å) and regular periods (550–600 Å). New collagen fibers (scar) will have variations in diameter and irregular arrangement. These fibrils are embedded in "ground substance" or glycosaminoglycans of which keratan sulfate is the most important. The sulfate fraction of these glycans can be labeled with an isotope to follow its fate in the normal and in the grafted cornea. The proteins to which these glycans are attached to are antigenic. These and the glycans form the proteoglycans. They are large molecules that tend to retain water. It is through these substances that nutrition reaches the keratocytes, and metabolic interchanges occur. The keratocytes are connective tissue cells located inside the collagen bundles (Fig. 2-2). Their cytoplasmic prolongations extend far from the cell body and make contact with other cells (Fig. 2-4). They respond to injury by becoming spindle shaped and mobilizing. In effect, they transform to fibroblasts, and they may reproduce at the edge of, or within, the injured area.

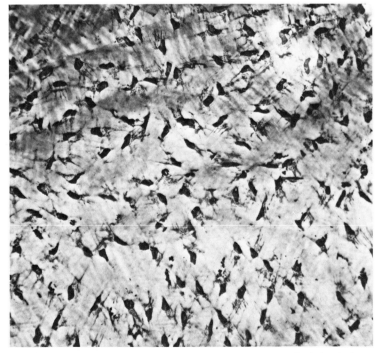

Figure 2-4. Human keratocytes in a keratoconus cornea. Cells join their cytoplasmic prolongations forming a syncitium (silver carbonate of del Rio Hortega, ×400).

Nerves

Corneal nerves lose their myelin cover once they enter the corneas; however, they retain their Schwann sheath. As soon as they enter the cornea, they branch into finer fibers (Fig. 2-5), and centrally, they form a plexus under the epithelium. They cross Bowman's membrane and fine twigs end between epithelial cells. These endings are sensitive to pain, pressure, and temperature.

Descemet's Membrane

This layer covers the posterior aspect of the cornea, and it is lined by endothelial (mesothelial) cells. These cells produce Descemet's membrane, a collagenous layer with a glycoprotein matrix. Ultramicroscopically, it has two regions: The anterior, which is banded, and the posterior, a nonbanded or homogenous region. In older corneas, this latter portion increases in thickness, but if excrescences or warts appear, as in Fuchs' dystrophy, then the collagen in the warts resembles that of the banded region. In spite of its apparent density, large molecules can diffuse through this layer into the stroma.

Endothelium

This is a single layer of hexagonal cells attached to Descemet's membrane by hemidesmosomes. Laterally, they are united by numerous interdigitations, desmosomal adhesions, and a *zonula occludens* on their surface. The number and size of cells vary with age. It is estimated that the normal adult cornea should

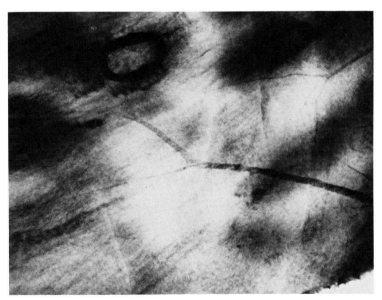

Figure 2-5. Nerves in the periphery of a rabbit cornea. Small branches start 2–3 mm inside the limbus (methylene blue, ×400).

have about 3000 cells/sq mm. Their surface shows microvilli (Fig. 2-6), and within their body, they show prominent endoplasmic reticulum, ribosomes, and long mitochondria. They all indicate that these cells are metabolically active, capable of synthetizing collagen, and maintaining the cornea deturgesced through their enzyme system.

A. THE SURVIVAL OF CELLULAR COMPONENTS

One of the most important problems in the field of tissue transplantation is that of host–donor interaction and the preservation of donor tissue identity after grafting. The information of donor tissue survival in corneal grafts was important to understand the behavior of transplants, because they contain the transplantational antigens. The survival of cells in corneal grafts was originally an academic question that could not be solved because suitable methods of identifying individual cells were not available. One such method became possible with the demonstration that ocular tissues could be labeled in an essentially permanent fashion by incorporation of tritiated thymidine into the nuclear DNA that was synthesized prior to division. Incorporation of this long-lived isotope in a stable biologic system of ocular tissue was first shown to occur in the lens after injury by Harding and his colleagues.[1] At about the same time, labeling of the corneal endothelium following injury was reported by Mills and Donn[2] and Bito and Harding.[3] In 1964, Polack[4] showed that this DNA label persisted in rabbit endothelium for at least 4 yr. Hanna and O'Brien[5] also demonstrated that thymidine could be incorporated by corneal stroma cells after intracorneal wounding with a blunt spatula. In 1962, Polack and Smelser[6-8] showed that stromal cells persisted in grafts for 1 yr and in the endothelium for at least 13 mo,[8] which was the end of the experiment. Hanna and Irwin also demonstrated

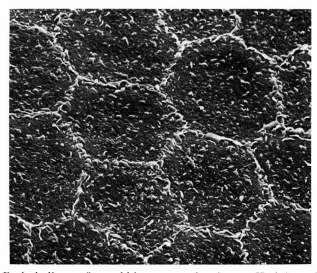

Figure 2-6. Endothelium of a rabbit cornea showing ruffled interdigitations and microvilli (SEM, ×5000).

in 1962 that endothelial cells survived in grafts for 13 mo.[9] It had been observed by Maumenee and Kornblueth[10] and Dunnington and Smelser[11] that freezing the central area of the cornea resulted in the death of all of the cells in this area that were replaced by mitosis and migration of cells from the unfrozen periphery. It was apparent then that using this method of corneal injury, stromal and endothelial cells could be labeled with tritiated thymidine at the time new DNA was synthesized. All daughter cells would contain this long-lived isotope, as shown for other cells.[12] This is essentially a permanent label, since corneal stroma and endothelial cells have a very low mitotic rate. In addition, this method would provide labeled cells homogenously distributed throughout the stroma and endothelial surface of the graft.

It was felt that the method of corneal cell labeling demonstrated by these experiments was superior to the method of sex chromatin labeling used by Basu et al.[13] and Espiritu et al.[14] and was more suitable for determining the degree of permanence of transplanted cells. The turnover rate for other corneal components, such as collagen and ground substance, is different from that of these cells and would be different in a corneal graft and therefore will be discussed in a different chapter.

Materials and Methods

LABELING OF DONOR TISSUE

Stroma cells. All corneal cells in a 6-mm central portion of rabbit corneas were destroyed by freezing with a 1 min application of a 5.5-mm conical cryocautery ($-79°C$). Four to six hours after freezing, corneal edema appeared that lasted for 4–5 days, after which the normal transparency of the cornea returned. The endothelium had regenerated by the sixth day without permanent damage to the collagen fibers, but stroma cell regenerations were slower. The regeneration of these cells was studied in a series of eyes removed 5 min, 4, 48, and 72 hr, and at 11, 21, and 100 days after freezing. The eyes were fixed in 10% formalin, the corneas removed, washed in tap water, and radial cuts made at their periphery so that they could be cut flat (tangentially). Frozen sections, 8–10 μ thick, were made and stained with the silver carbonate technique of del Rio Hortega[15] or with hematoxylin and eosin.

In another group of rabbits, regenerating cells were labeled by injecting into the anterior chamber 0.1 cc (2 μcm) of tritiated thymidine (sp./a 0.36 c/mM) dissolved in Eagle's basal medium. The labeled cells in the frozen sections were identified in radioautographs prepared by the stripping film method of Pelc[63] (Fig. 2-7).

Results showed that 5 min after freezing, the stromal cells appeared to be normal in appearance, but 4 hr later, when stromal edema had occurred, the central portion of the cornea contained only grossly abnormal cells or silver-stained cellular debris. In general, the central area was well delineated from the peripheral cornea that contained normal-appearing keratoblasts. Mitotic figures appeared at 48 hr at the edge of the injury. On the third day, the previously frozen zone was partially repopulated by fibroblastic cells that formed a

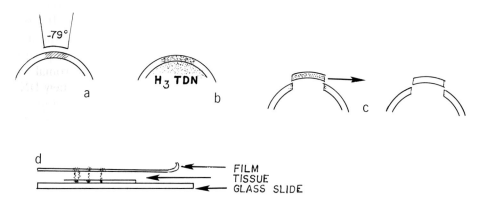

Figure 2-7. Drawing illustrating **A.** the destruction of corneal cells with a cryocautery, and **B.** corneal labeling by intracameral injections of thymidine. **C.** Labeled corneas are grafted to unlabeled recipients. **D.** Sections of labeled tissue are coated with photographic film for radioautography.

palisade-like ring, many of which appeared to be migrating towards the central corneal area among several polymorphonuclear leukocytes.

One week later, the injured cornea contained a few cells, which greatly increased in number by the end of the second week. Most of these cells still did not have the appearance of typical keratoblasts, but by the third week, the central area was almost completely filled by fibroblasts, most of which were throwing out lateral processes and assuming the appearance of normal keratoblasts. Corneas examined 6 mo after freezing showed almost complete repopulation of the central cornea with corneal cells, with a few less differentiated fibroblasts.

When daily single injections of ^{3}H-thymidine were made into the anterior chamber of eyes frozen 1–7 days earlier, the labeled cells formed a ring approximately the size of the previously frozen area. Labeled cells were found mostly in the central part of the cornea when the injections were done at 5–7 days. Six weeks later, labeled cells were found only in the central cornea, but they were fewer in number than when injections were done early.

We found that daily injections of ^{3}H-thymidine during an 8-day period after freezing produced the best label, which eventually was homogenously distributed in the central cornea. Approximately 10%–15% of the stromal cells in this area were well labeled, and this label persisted for over 12 mo (Fig. 2-8).

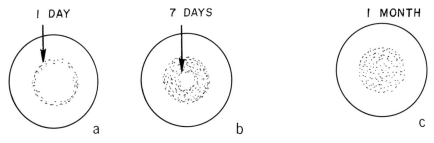

Figure 2-8. ^{3}H-thymidine labeling of stromal cells **A.** 1 day after freezing, **B.** after seven injections, and **C.** 1 mo later.

Endothelial cells.   Single injections of ³H-thymidine (2 μCi) in the anterior chamber of eyes with frozen corneas resulted in inadequate labeling, because the injected thymidine was rapidly eliminated from the anterior chamber. Therefore, as for stromal labeling, repeated daily injections were required, in this case for the first 5 days after freezing (Fig. 2-9).

A month was allowed to elapse between the last thymidine injection and transplantation, thus permitting complete recovery of the cornea from the trauma of freezing and labeling, as well as the complete removal of nonincorporated isotope.

Epithelial cells..   Corneal epithelial cells were labeled by frequent (5 times a day) instillations of ³H-thymidine (2 μCi) or an ointment containing approximately 2 μCi per application (4 times a day). The labeling procedure was continued for a period of 1 wk, and 10%–20% of basal cells were labeled in this fashion. The labeling however, decreased by 50% in another week by cell turnover, thus making this system unsuitable for the study of epithelial cell survival in corneal grafts.

SURGICAL PROCEDURE

Albino rabbits (2.5–3.0 kg) were used as hosts and donors, and partial (4.5 or 5 mm) penetrating keratoplasties were made using the labeled donor material. The technique of graft fixation with splint sutures in order to minimize graft damage was described in chapter 1. Fifty percent crystal-clear grafts were obtained. Cloudy, infected, or dislocated grafts were discarded, but about 10% of grafts that were slightly hazy or edematous at the time of suture removal were also studied.

These labeled grafts were removed at periods ranging from 1 wk to 13 mo and then processed for autoradiography.

Results

THE FATE OF STROMAL CELLS

Tritium-labeled cells were found to persist in nongrafted corneas (controls) for as long as 35 mo. Labeled donor cells were found in 11 of 12 transparent grafts. Seven of these were studied at 12–13 mo after keratoplasty, and they

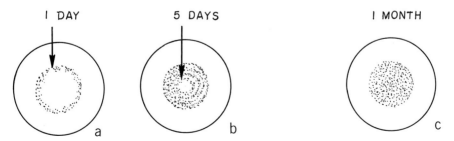

Figure 2-9.   Uptake of ³H-thymidine by regenerating endothelium **A.** 1 day, **B.** after five injections of the isotope, and **C.** at the end of 1 mo.

contained labeled donor cells (Fig. 2-10). No trace of original donor cells could be found in seven hazy grafts nor in five that had become clear after early haziness at 12 mo. However, donor keratocytes survived in two grafts (3.5- and 8-mo-old) that had been turbid but had regained transparency.

THE FATE OF CORNEAL ENDOTHELIUM

The endothelium of 27 corneal grafts, ranging in age from 1 wk to 13 mo, were studied. Labeled (donor) endothelial cells were found in 19 clear grafts, including 4 12-mo-old grafts (Figs. 2-11 and 2-12). Two clear grafts produced unsatisfactory autoradiographs. The endothelium of three transplants, which had at one time been hazy but recovered before autopsy, contained no isotopic labeling. None of three opaque grafts contained labeled endothelial cells, indicating that they had been completely replaced by unlabeled host cells.

The intensity of labeling of individual cells ranged from "dense," that is, heavy blackening of the emulsion, to a relatively light scattering of silver grains over the nucleus. In general, the intensity of cell labeling in older grafts was not appreciably less than that of younger grafts.

THE FATE OF EPITHELIAL CELLS

The turnover rate of these cells did not allow us to follow the fate of labeled cells longer than 1 wk after keratoplasty. About 10% of labeled cells were present in grafts and in the epithelial plug at the host–graft junction. Two weeks after keratoplasty, autoradiographs were negative.

Discussion

The results of these experiments demonstrated that grafted stromal and endothelial cells, in the absence of graft damage or rejection, may persist almost indefinitely and confirm clinical evidence of grafts clear for several years on corneas affected with Fuchs' dystrophy. These results were in agreement with reports of Hanna et al.[5] and with the studies of Basu et al.,[4,13] who, using sex chromatin as a marker, found that homografted stromal cells persisted for 3 mo. Espiritu et al.,[14] also using the sex chromatin method, found that transplanted endothelial cells persisted for several months, but replacement of donor cells by host cells seemed to occur after 5–7 mo. This difference with our results was

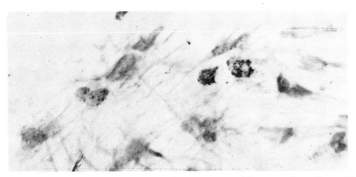

Figure 2-10.   Labeled keratocytes in a 12-mo-old corneal graft (×400).

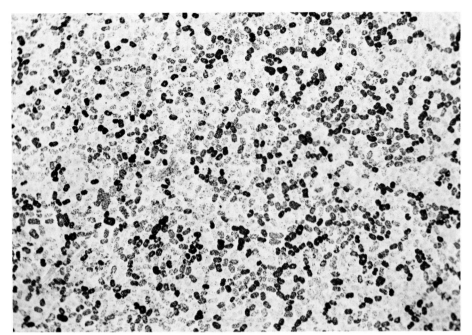

Figure 2-11. High-power view of labeled endothelium prior to transplantation. There is 100% label (×120).

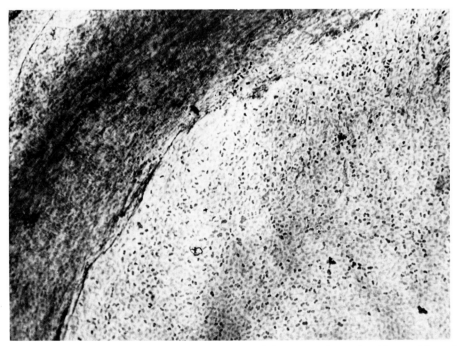

Figure 2-12. Radioautograph of a flat endothelial preparation of a 12-mo-old graft. Labeled cells persist to the edge of the graft and partially cover the scar (×50).

probably due to too few cases studied by Espiritu et al. and technical difficulties with their method of cell tracing.

Dohlman[16] earlier attempted to follow the fate of transplanted donor cells by labeling them with ^{32}P. His experiments suggested a rapid replacement of the grafted cells; however, ^{32}P is not incorporated exclusively in stable tissue constituents, which may explain the rapid decrease in the isotope that he found. In addition, the physical half-life of this isotope is too short for the long-term experiments required by this problem.

Thymidine labeling of donor cells has the advantage of ready identification, since ^{3}H-thymidine is incorporated in a stable cellular component (DNA) and does not exchange with the thymidine of other cells or with the body fluids during the life of the cell. It does, however, subject the labeled cell to some radiation, but this was believed to be insignificant and an unimportant factor in these experiments, since any damage that the cells might sustain should decrease, rather than prolong, their life after transplantation. There is good reason to believe that the unlabeled host corneal cells cannot acquire an isotopic label from the graft. Relatively large amounts of ^{3}H-thymidine are required to label corneal cells, the excess of which disappears completely and quickly after injection.[17,18] The isotopic label that might be released by the death of a labeled cell would be far too small to relabel other cells, because it would be immediately diluted in the tissue fluid and excreted. Furthermore, in order to incorporate such released isotope, the unlabeled cell would have to be engaged in DNA synthesis at precisely that moment, which is unlikely, since the rate of cell division of corneal stroma and endothelium is extremely low. No evidence of labeling of host keratoblasts in or near the scar was found; however, the possibility of reuse of the isotopical label by corneal cells was investigated in other experiments, and no transfer of label was detected.[17]

The intensity of the autographs (number of silver grains in the emulsion over the nuclei and the number of labeled cells) was less in the stroma than in the endothelium. This was due in part to a longer regeneration period of stromal cells, the intermittent label with ^{3}H-thymidine, and the fact that the weak beta particles of tritium have an average path in tissue of about 1.0 μ; as a result, the photographic emulsion was affected only by radioactive nuclei present in the superficial portion of the 8.0-μ section. Nuclei slightly deeper in the sections would appear to contain little isotope, because only a few of the emitted beta particles could reach the emulsion, and nuclei lying still deeper would not affect the emulsion at all.[18] In contrast, all of the endothelial nuclei are in one layer and sufficiently near the emulsion to produce a sharp radioautographic image.

Donor cells were not found in several months old, permanently opaque grafts and rarely in those which had transient edema and recovered transparency. Hanna,[9] however, found labeled cells in 10-day-old, partially dislocated, cloudy grafts. Also, Klen and Hradil[19] found donor cells, identified by sex chromatin, in opaque 12- and 32-mo-old grafts removed from two patients at the time of retransplantation, but the authors did not mention the number or proportion of donor-to-host cells found.

The absence of labeled (stromal and endothelial) cells in opaque grafts and in those with a transitory opacification suggests that host cells had replaced those of the graft without necessarily affecting its transparency, unless the graft became vascularized and invaded with scar tissue. Usually, graft haziness indicates death of donor endothelial cells, and its subsequent clearing suggests that new cells had repopulated the graft or surviving cells recovered areas of damage. In such cases of transient haziness, vascularization and inflammation was absent or minimal, and graft invasion by host fibroblasts did not occur.

We cannot assume that the behavior of donor cells in these experimental grafts necessarily duplicates that which occurs in the human, because absolutely fresh donor corneas were grafted into normal recipients with a minimum of graft trauma, since these were secured only by splint sutures. The situation is different with Eye Bank eyes where we find that endothelial cells have changes related to aging and various degrees of damage when stored in moist chambers at 4°C (see chapter 16). We believe that cutting the graft with scissors, plus its necessary manipulation while edge-to-edge suturing is being done, probably results in the death of large numbers of endothelial as well as stromal cells at the graft margins.[20] Recent investigations with the specular microscope of Maurice suggest that human graft endothelial cells enlarge tremendously to cover areas of cell destruction rather than being replaced by many small cells.[20] In 1967, Salceda[33] showed that the endothelium of experimental grafts (chromatin label) persisted for months. Clear grafts were obtained from donor tissue as old as 21 days (4°C) as long as it had 50% of donor cells.

Scar tissue is primarily of host origin, including the endothelium covering the scar. Only in one specimen, we found a continuous sheet of donor endothelial cells covering the scar and a small portion of the host where the endothelium had, no doubt, been injured at the time of transplantation. The extreme freshness of donor tissue probably accounted for this finding. The information that scar tissue originates mostly from the host has been confirmed by Kuwabara[22] and is most valuable if we consider that corneas with chronic edema heal poorly, because they have fewer and abnormal corneal cells. It appears, therefore, that the varied opinions of earlier workers on cell survival of corneal transplants were only partially correct. This subject has been well reviewed and discussed by Castroviejo[23] and Geeraets.[24] Maumenee and Kornblueth[25] and Paufique and Offret,[26] for example, suggested that some of the transplanted cells may survive. Magitot[27] also thought survival was possible, and Babel[28] and Katzin and Kuo,[29] on the other hand, felt that final replacement of donor cells by host cells occurred, but that the noncellular donor stroma persisted.

Each corneal component need not persist to the same degree when transplanted. Tritium-labeled epithelial cells were found to survive at least 5 days following transplantation. The thymidine-labeling technique is not well suited to the study of the persistence of these cells because their rapid rate of mitosis dilutes the label until it cannot be detected. However, using the sex chromatin technique, Arkin et al.[30] observed that the donor epithelium of corneal grafts in rabbits was replaced by the host after the seventh day. This finding is not supported by the experiments of Khodadoust and Silverstein who demonstrated long-term survival of certain number of epithelial cells in allografts[31] and even in heterografts[32] if the immune reaction is controlled. The experiments reported here demonstrate that stromal and endothelial cells may persist indefinitely when transplanted, although this survival is affected by the freshness of the donor tissue and the surgical trauma. The low incidence of immune reactions in avascular host corneas is another factor favoring long-term survival of donor tissue.

It is possible that the freeze-injured donor tissue may have developed a subendothelial fibrous membrane.[34] The donor endothelial tissue, however, had normal morphology and function. The corneas were clear, controls retained the label for 4 yr, and 70% of grafts remained clear for several months.

The clinical demonstration of endothelial cell survival in transplants is observed in successful grafts for corneal edema. These can remain clear for many years.

B. THE SURVIVAL OF NONCELLULAR COMPONENTS

Collagen

Collagen, long considered a nonliving component of the cornea, is a biochemically active substance constantly in the process of synthesis and remolding by the action of enzymes. The turnover of collagen, however, is very slow,[35-37] so much that its half-life is probably as long as the life of the experimental animal. We assumed that the corneal collagen should also share this low turnover, even after transplantation, because we had seen that cellular components persisted for long periods of time in corneal grafts. As in previous studies with isotopic labeling of donor tissue, the amino acids forming the alpha chains of collagen could be isotopically labeled to trace this substance as we had done with the cells. In these studies, glycine was isotopically labeled with carbon-14 and administered to young animals (who were rapidly synthesizing collagen). The rate of collagen synthesis and destruction by collagenases decreases in the older animal; however, since this turnover is slow and the half-life of the isotope is long, we could follow the transplanted collagen by radioautographic methods for long periods of time. Our studies showed that the label persisted in grafts for several months with almost no change in its density.

MATERIALS AND METHODS

Experiment I. Labeling of collagen tissue required that young albino rabbits, 3–4-wk-old (1500–2000 g) receive 0.4 μCi of ^{14}C-glycine (0.10 cc) subconjunctivally three times a week for a total of 12 injections (4.8 μCi/cornea). The injections were made at different locations around the limbus so that an even circumlimbal infiltration of the labeled amino acid was accomplished in an effort to obtain an homogenous distribution within the cornea. Since it has been shown that isotopic glycine is first incorporated into soluble collagen and noncollagen proteins,[38] the labeled corneas were not used for 2½ mo after the last injection to allow conversion of the soluble to insoluble collagen and reduction by metabolic turnover of other isotopically labeled soluble proteins. At that time, 5-mm grafts were made from labeled donor corneas to nonlabeled hosts. The remainder of each donor cornea was spread flat, assisted by a few radial incisions at the limbus, dried between two pieces of polyvinylidine film (Saran, Dow Chemical Co., sold as Saran-Wrap®),[39] and preserved in this fashion for future radioautography.

Nineteen grafts were made; 15 of these were clear, and 4 were hazy. Studies were made at periods of time varying from 8 to 17 mo postgrafting. At autopsy, the grafted corneas were mounted flat between Saran sheets and dried (Fig. 2-13).

The grafted and donor corneas were then mounted together and placed between two 1 × 3-inch Kodak radioautographic plates for exposure. This made comparison of the intensity of the autograph of the donor cornea and graft possible on the same plate.

Experiment II. These were done to secure data necessary to support the essential questions asked in these experiments: Namely, does the collagen of the

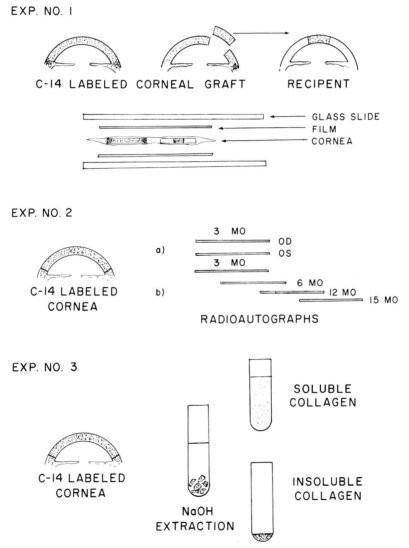

Figure 2-13. Persistence of collagen in corneal grafts: the three experimental procedures used to determine the fate of transplanted collagen.

cornea persist when grafted, and are the radioautographic methods reliable for securing this information? Other corneas labeled with ^{14}C-glycine, as before, were also prepared for radioautography to show: (A) the variations in the degree of labeling secured and (B) the degree of retention of the isotopic label when the cornea was not transplanted. In experiment (A), the corneas of both eyes were labeled. Three months later, both eyes were removed and autographs made, so that differences in the amount of ^{14}C-glycine administered, or the efficiency of its incorporation by the two corneas, could be compared. In experiment (B), the labeled corneas were prepared for autography 3 mo after the last isotope injection. Other animals were kept for an additional 12 mo (15 mo after the last ^{14}C-glycine injection) to determine whether a change occurred during this period.

All of the autographs that were compared in any one experiment had been exposed to the radioactive tissue for the same period of time and had developed simultaneously; therefore, the length of exposure and the photographic process were constant. All of the radioautographs were then placed side by side in contact with a sheet of photographic film and a negative made of all of them simultaneously. Therefore, the density of any autographs shown could be compared to another with assurance that no variation due to the procedures mentioned above had affected their density.

Experiment III. This series of experiments was performed to determine what proportion of the radioactivity, demonstrated in autographs, was due to the isotopic label in collagen rather than in the noncollagen portions of the cornea. Twenty-two young rabbit corneas were labeled as before, and either 24 days, 9 wks, or 3 mo after the last injection, the animals were autopsied, the corneas dissected carefully, and stored frozen until the collagen and noncollagen fractions could be separated and their radioactivity determined, (Fig. 2-13, Exp. III). Their insoluble (collagen) and soluble (noncollagen) fractions were separated by the method used by Herrmann and Barry[40] based on that of Lowry et al.[41] The frozen corneas, each of which weighed about 50.0 mg, were thawed, separately finely minced with scissors, ground in heavy walled test tubes with four parts sand to one part cornea (by weight) in 0.05 M sodium hydroxide at 4°C, and centrifuged. Three 2-hr and one short (few minutes) sodium hydroxide extractions were made with frequent stirring, regrinding in the cold, and centrifugation. The supernatant solutions were pooled. The residue of insoluble material (collagen) was dissolved in distilled water by autoclaving for 1.5 hr at 18-lb pressure. After autoclaving, the solution was separated from the sand by centrifuge, the process repeated to ascertain that no insoluble corneal tissue remained in the sand, and the two clear autoclaved supernatant fractions pooled. Additional extractions with autoclaving showed that the collagen had been dissolved. The radioactivity of both the soluble (noncollagen) and insoluble (collagen) fractions was determined with a Packard scintillation counter.

RESULTS

Experiment I. Autographs of two of nine corneal grafts and of the donor cornea from which they were taken are shown in Figure 2-14. The ages of the grafts ranged from 6-17 mo, and all except one were clear transplants. Compari-

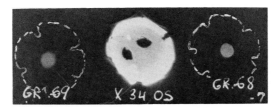

Figure 2-14. Radioautograph of ^{14}C-labeled grafts, 6 mo (GR 69) and 10 mo (GR 68) following keratoplasty. Control cornea in center shows slightly more radioactivity.

son of the intensity of the autographs of the donor and transplanted tissue reveals very little difference between them, indicating retention of donor label. The edges of autographs of the transplants were sharp, with no indication that the isotopic label was transferred from the donor to the host or into the tissue at the edge of the graft, which was the site of active collagen breakdown and synthesis during scar formation. The autograph of the one hazy transplant showed a marked loss of donor label.

Experiment II.   The persistence of the ^{14}C-glycine component in nongrafted corneas was essentially similar in corneas removed at 3, 6, and 12 mo. The 15-mo-old cornea showed slightly less intensity in the autograph. Some of this difference could be due to the amount of isotope originally administered or incorporated into the cornea. The variation, which can be expected due to this factor, was negligible as determined in a series of radioautographs of right and left eyes of the same animal labeled 3 mo previously.

Experiment III.   Radioassay of the collagen and noncollagen fractions of 22 corneas showed that after only 24 days, about 90% of the radioactivity was found in the collagen fraction (Fig. 2-15). The proportion of radioactivity of the soluble noncollagen fraction in the 9-wk and the 3-mo group decreased still further, mostly due to reduction of the noncollagen fraction. At 3 mo, nearly 97% of the isotopic label was confined to the collagen fraction.[45]

DISCUSSION

A portion of the collagen of nearly all tissues consists of a soluble hydroxyproline-containing protein, a "soluble collagen." The amount of this soluble collagen is greater in growing animals than in older and nongrowing ones.[42,43] Collagen, when first synthesized by the fibroblast, presumably is in soluble form and is later converted to the insoluble type (see chapter 4, Fig. 4-22). Therefore, some of the soluble ^{14}C-labeled material that was found, especially at 24 days (Fig. 2-15), may have been soluble collagen. However, all the autographs shown are of corneas at least 3 mo after the last ^{14}C-glycine injection and, therefore, would indicate that almost all the labeled collagen was of the insoluble type and only 3%–4% was soluble material. Advantage was taken of the rapid synthesis of collagen in the growing animal to secure an appreciable final incorporation of the isotopic label in the insoluble, more stable fraction.

It does not appear likely that the ^{14}C-glycine label in the collagen was exchanged with the glycine pool, because there was no evidence of the diffusion of

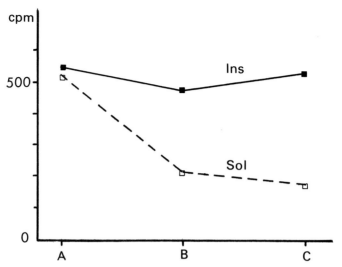

Figure 2-15. ^{14}C-glycine content on corneal insoluble collagen (Ins) and soluble collagen (Sol). The ratio of insoluble to soluble collagen gradually increases (**A**, 24 days; **B**, 9 wk; **C**, 3 mo; (reproduced by permission.[11])

the isotopic label from the grafts to be incorporated in the host cornea or in the rapidly growing scar. The possibility of such a label exchange has been suggested by Robertson.[44] Some small rate of turnover of even the stable collagens of the skin and tendon have been assumed to exist.[35,37]

Radioautography was chosen as the method of analysis of this problem because the small amount of tissue in a corneal graft would make accurate counting procedures questionable. In addition, radioautography would reveal any heterogeneity in the distribution of the label (e.g., at the edge of the scar where some destruction of donor and host tissue would conceivably take place). An objection to the autographic method is the difficulty in the quantitative interpretation. This was solved by placing the autographs of donor and graft close to each other on a single autographic plate and by preparing the reproduction of them in a manner minimizing photographic variables. Some slight reduction in autographic density of the grafts, relative to the donor corneas, may be indicated in a few of the autographs. These differences were comparable to those of the 3- and 15-mo nongrafted corneas. Therefore, although some turnover of collagen in grafts may exist, it is certainly slight and does not proceed at a greater rate than normal.

Analysis of the radioactivity of collagen and noncollagen fractions of the cornea show that almost all (96%–97%) of the isotopic label was in insoluble collagen at the time the grafts were made,[45] and therefore, we may conclude that the autographs represent essentially nothing but that corneal constituent. A considerable change in intensity was seen in autographs (not figured) of corneas taken shortly (1 mo) after the glycine had been administered and in others prepared 3 mo later, which indicated that incorporation of the isotopic label in a stable tissue constituent is a relatively slow process, appearing to be essentially complete in 2–3 mo.

All of the studies on the persistence of donor tissue components in corneal grafts indicate that they are not replaced at a rate appreciably greater than is characteristic in unoperated corneas. This observation, however, may not apply to the perimeter of the graft, which is subject to damage during surgery.

The experiments reported here lead us to the conclusion that the stromal collagen of a corneal graft is largely the original donor material and is not changed appreciably after transplantation for a period at least as long as 17 mo, provided the graft is healthy and remains transparent. Hazy grafts, in contrast, undergo relatively rapid removal and/or synthesis of new collagen.

The Turnover of Ground Substance

As previously described, proteoglycans form a large portion of the interfibrillar substance of the cornea. This substance is made by the keratocytes, and therefore, it was natural to attempt to study the survival of stroma cells after keratoplasty indirectly, by determining the production of corneal mucopolysaccharides (MP). Earlier work by Bostrom[46] and Bostrom and Gardell[47] show that when inorganic ^{35}S is administered to an animal, the isotope is incorporated by MPs in all parts of the body. In the eye, the uptake of ^{35}S by cornea and sclera was shown by Odeblad and Bostrom,[48] by Dohlman and Bostrom,[49] and by Dohlman.[50]

The in vitro ^{35}S incorporation by keratocytes of corneal grafts was studied by Dohlman in 1957.[51] In one experiment, he performed 6-mm grafts in rabbits, and at different periods of time after keratoplasty, the transplants were removed. The grafts were then incubated in ^{35}S NaSO$_4$ for 4 hr, washed, dried, and the radioactivity counted. He found that there was a low uptake of ^{35}S by corneal cells in the first 2 wk postsurgery. Thereafter, the uptake was slightly more than that of the control corneas. Radioautographic studies of corneas following keratoplasty showed that uptake was greater at the scar site.

In another study,[52] Dohlman grafted donor corneas labeled 3 days previously with ^{35}S and determined the loss of radioactivity in grafts removed at various days after keratoplasty. Controls were nongrafted labeled corneas. These experiments showed that in the corneal transplants, the radioactivity decreased faster than in the normal cornea during the first 2 wk following transplantation. After this initial loss of radioactivity, the elimination of ^{35}S occurred at the same rate in the graft as in the normal control corneas (Fig. 2-16). Similar experiments were done by LaTessa in 1960.[53] This author tried to determine the rate and the route of ^{35}S elimination from the graft. He also found that the 7-day-old graft had 66% of ^{35}S as compared to controls, and 40%, 2 wk after keratoplasty. These figures are slightly lower than those reported by Dohlman, but they both concluded that there was a faster elimination of the labeled ground substance immediately following keratoplasty. LaTessa indicated that the radioactive sulfate was probably eliminated through the anterior chamber and the corneal surface, since no significant sulfate was detected in the unlabeled host corneas.

In experiments we performed where we injected ^{35}S-labeled sodium sulfate in the anterior chamber of eyes containing corneal grafts, we found that the radioactivity of the ground substance of the graft was similar to that of the host

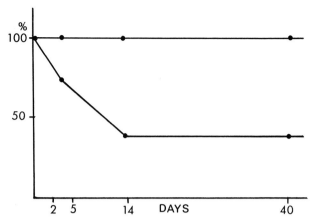

Figure 2-16. Graph showing the loss of ^{35}S-labeled sulfated mucopolysaccharides in corneal grafts at various days following transplantation. (Reproduced by permission.[52])

cornea, as determined by radioautographs, (see Figure 4-6, chapter 4). It should be mentioned, however, that the uptake of ^{35}S by host cornea was also decreased, as shown by Dohlman and LaTessa. When we compared these corneas to the labeled normal cornea, we found no significant difference in radioactivity by radioautography. This technique probably is not sensitive enough to detect a 40% or 50% drop in radioactivity as shown by the abovementioned investigators. Also, the decreased uptake of ^{35}S by recent corneal grafts and its adjacent host tissue may be related to edema of the corneal stroma as a result of surgical trauma.[54,55]

Since our investigations have shown that corneal stromal cells persist in the graft for long periods of time following transplantation, we must consider two possibilities: (1) that these cells continue with their normal production of proteoglycans with an apparent decrease of the labeled substance due to edema or (2) that there is a large destruction of keratocytes in the graft due to surgical trauma. Since edema of the graft and the host cornea is characteristic of penetrating grafts for the first 10 days following keratoplasty, we may assume that this is the cause of the ^{35}S loss from tissues labeled before grafting and the decreased uptake of the isotope by transplants following keratoplasty.

The Regeneration of Corneal Nerves

Corneal transplants do not require the regeneration of nerves for their incorporation and to obtain normal transparency. On a long-term basis, however, grafts deprived of innervation frequently develop epithelial defects and ulcerations. The regeneration of corneal nerves following keratoplasty is related to the presence of normal nerve branches prior to keratoplasty. It has been estimated by Escapini[56] that, on the average, corneal transplants require 90 days to obtain sensation. In patients with keratoconus or central corneal scars and normal peripheral corneal sensitivity, we have been able to confirm this period of time; however, in corneas with more structural changes or with severe herpetic disease, the recovery of sensitivity may be more delayed or never attained. In experimental corneal grafts, Escapini found that there were signs of regeneration of nerve branches in the host cornea following keratoplasty. Regeneration of these nerves occurred along the scar tissue first and then into the corneal transplant itself.

Rexed and Rexed[57] observed nerve degeneration 7 days following corneal section in the rabbit, with regeneration beginning 3 days later. Zander and Wedell[58] also found nerves of viable appearance 7 days after similar lesions and in keratoplasty. New nerve fibers were distinguished mainly by their thinness and tortuous pathways. In successive days, new fibers increased in thickness.

Corroborating our clinical experience, Rexed[59] found that graft innervation occurred whether the graft was clear or opaque. However, this is difficult to demonstrate because corneal sensitivity is decreased in corneas with abnormal epithelium or with epithelial edema.

C. THE FATE OF STROMA CELLS IN HETEROLOGOUS CORNEAL GRAFTS

It has been shown that cells of successful corneal grafts obtained from an animal of the same species (allografts) may persist indefinitely, and therefore, true chimeras may be produced. Evidence suggests that, to a great extent, the high success of these grafts is due to its avascular character, since grafts in vascularized hosts lose that privilege. The situation is different for penetrating transplants obtained from animals of different species (xenografts), because

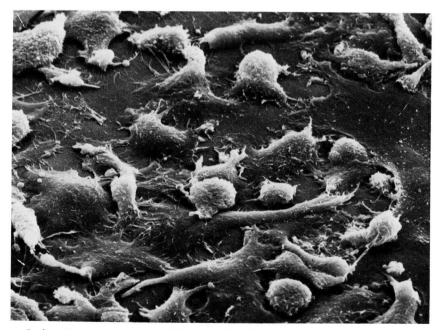

Figure 2-17.   Human corneal graft in the rabbit depicting endothelial rejection. Numerous endothelial cells have been destroyed baring Descemet's membrane. Several lymphocytes are present in this area of rejection (SEM, ×2500).

even if placed in avascular host corneas, they are rejected. This rejection may be caused by the greater antigenic response engendered by foreign tissue. The more distant host and donor are from the zoologic scale, the more rapid and violent the graft rejection is; the cornea, however, appears to be a privileged site with respect to lamellar heterologous transplants. Fully penetrating corneal xenografts are rejected between 2 and 4 wk (Fig. 2-17), but lamellar or intralamellar xenografts may persist for long periods of time. The survival of these grafts raised the question of whether their cells died shortly after grafting and what remained was the nonliving stromal tissue that possibly could be repopulated by stroma cells. This question was investigated by Basu and Sarkar[60] by placing cat corneas, wrapped in plastic film and Millipore filter (to prevent contact of host cells with the donor tissue), between the corneal lamellas of rabbits. They found that the heterologous cells, identified by chromosome analysis, survived at least 43 days. Algire[61] has shown that these filters form an effective barrier that prevents host cells from reaching a graft and causing its rejection. However, the question of survival of heterologous cells in corneal grafts, where they are in intimate contact with the host, remained unanswered. In 1964, we[62] studied the survival of isotopically labeled cells of intralamellar heterologous corneal transplants and found that these cells persisted for many months as long as the graft remained clear and avascular.

Materials and Methods

The central 6 mm of rabbit corneas were frozen for 1 min by the application of a cryocautery ($-79°C$). As in previous studies, the injured area was labeled by injecting tritiated thymidine (2 μCi) into the anterior chamber, daily, for the first 5 days after freezing. From 20% to 25% of stroma cells were demonstrably labeled in the regenerated area. The eyes were allowed to recover from this process for 1 mo, in order to permit complete repopulation of the central cornea by isotopically labeled cells and the removal of all tritiated thymidine that had not been incorporated in the DNA. Intralamellar transplants of full-thickness labeled rabbit corneas, 4.5 mm in diameter, were then made into cat corneas.

Cat eyes bearing grafts were removed at 2, 3, 4½, 8, 10, and 10½ mo. The corneas were fixed in formaldehyde, and frozen sections tangential to the surface of the cornea were cut off some of the transplants. Other corneas were embedded in paraffin and 5-μ sections cut perpendicular to the corneal surface. Radioautographs were prepared of both the paraffin and frozen sections by the method of Pelc.[65]

Results

Four eyes with clear grafts were sectioned 2–3 mo after transplantation, and the number of labeled cells in the grafts was found to be essentially the same as in labeled nongrafted corneas, i.e., 20% labeled cells. However, grafts from 4½ mo of age and older contained only 10% of labeled donor cells. The total number as well as the percentage of labeled cells was still less (2%–5%) in grafts 8 and 10 mo old. No labeled cells were found in the 10½-mo-old grafts. Four 2-mo-old grafts that became opaque and vascular showed no labeled donor cells. Two control intralamellar allografts (10½ mo) showed persistence of over 20% labeled donor cells (Table 1).

Table 1

Persistence of Donor Keratocytes in Xenografts

Graft No.	Age of Graft (mo)	Survival of Donor Keratocytes	Condition of Graft
Heterografts			
1	2	+++	Clear
2	2	+++	Clear
3	2	0	Opaque, vascular
4	2	0	Opaque, vascular
5	2	0	Opaque, vascular
6	2	0	Opaque, vascular
7	3	+++	Clear
8	3	+++	Clear
9	4½	++	Clear
10	4½	++	Clear
11	8¼	+	Clear
12	10	+	Clear
13	10½	0	Clear
Homografts			
14	10½	++	Clear
15	10½	+	Clear

+++, Approximately 20% of labeled cells throughout the graft. Most are heavily labeled.

++, Approximately 10% of labeled cells throughout the graft. Some are heavily labeled. Most are moderately labeled.

+, Approximately 2%–5% of labeled cells through the graft, with an occasional cell heavily labeled, a few moderately labeled, others faintly labeled.

0, No evidence of surviving donor cells.

Five intralamellar allografts were made of labeled, but dead (killed by repeated freezing and thawing), rabbit corneas. Radioautografts of the host corneas were uniformly negative, indicating that host cells failed to incorporate the small amount of isotopic label from the debris of labeled grafts. Autographs of the dead donor tissue were positive, showing that tritiated material was present.

Discussion

These experiments demonstrated that cells of xenografts can survive for long periods of time as long as the host is avascular; however, these results depended on the assumption that the label lost by donor cells is not reutilized by cells of the host. In earlier studies[64] on the fate of labeled keratoblasts in homo-transplants, it was noted that the host cells adjacent to the graft did not become labeled, although undoubtably, cell division had occurred in this region when materials derived from dead labeled cells at the edge of the transplant were available. Scullica et al.[65] found that labeled nuclear material in the lens, released when the cells were destroyed by irradiation, was not reutilized to any significant extent by rapidly dividing nearby cells. However, Bryant[66] injected thymidine-labeled leukocytes in partially hepatectomized mice and reported that a small percentage (0.5%–1.0%) of the hepatic cells became labeled. For this reason, some of the experiments reported here are of special importance. By making intralamellar implants containing labeled, but dead, keratocytes (frozen), the host cells were stimulated to divide by the injury of the operation. No evidence of reutilization of the labeled nuclear debris was obtained, either in these experiments or in those in which regenerating endothelial cells were exposed to homogenized labeled dead tissue injected or implanted in the anterior chamber. These experiments strongly supported the conclusion that the labeled cells found in the heterografts originated in the donor and were not host cells labeled with the isotope released from the graft.

Most of the experiments on heterologous intralamellar corneal transplants have demonstrated persistence of the graft as a whole and as a transparent tissue; but it was not shown that these grafts either contained living cells or, if they did, that they were not host cells that had invaded the transplant subsequent to the death of the donor cells. Our experiments showed that the keratoblasts of intralamellar corneal xenografts maintain themselves in the cornea of another species for an astonishingly long period of time. The persistence of heterologous cells in the cornea may very well be due to the avascular quality of the tissue and to the small mass of heterologous tissue that is introduced into the host. Such grafts, if small, may be an inadequate antigenic stimulus, particularly when placed in a host cornea where, without vascular or lymphatic connections, the opportunity for foreign antigens to come in contact with host antibody-producing cells is greatly reduced. In addition, should even a weak antigen reaction be produced, the avascular, alymphatic bed of the graft that completely surrounds it may very well inhibit the delivery of cell-borne antibodies to the graft. Very antigenic donor tissue (distant in zoologic scale) can stimulate vascularization even if small in size. In this event, the "privileged" characteristic of the cornea would disappear. It does not seem likely that the avascularity of the cornea would protect the graft from soluble antibodies, because host proteins of this size (as those from the graft) should diffuse without difficulty throughout the corneal stroma.[67] In general, humoral antibodies and complement do not participate in graft rejections, but our inability to detect them does not negate their presence. The decrease in the number of donor keratocytes could have been due to these circulating antibodies or to continued replication of these cells with eventual loss of their label. Intralamellar grafts enjoy more protection than penetrating grafts, because these have their endothelial layer exposed to aqueous humor and to leukocytes of uveal origin. Rejection of heterologous penetrating grafts occurs violently in the endothelial layer, while the same tissue placed intralamellarly may not be rejected.

REFERENCES

1. Harding CV, Donn A, Srinivasan BD: Incorporation of thymidine by injured lens epithelium. Exp Eye Res 18:582, 1959
2. Mills NL, Donn A: Incorporation of tritium-labeled thymidine by rabbit corneal endothelium, *In* Smelser GK (ed): Structure of the Eye. New York, Academic, 1961, pp 435–439

3. Bito LZ, Harding CV: Tritium retention by corneal endothelium after incorporation of H³-thymidine. Arch Ophthalmol 65:553, 1961
4. Polack FM: Four year retention of H-thymidine by corneal endothelium. Arch Ophthalmol 75:659, 1966
5. Hanna C, O'Brien JE: Thymidine-tritium labeling of the cellular elements of the corneal stroma. Arch Ophthalmol 66:362, 1961
6. Polack FM, Smelser GK: The persistence of isotopically labeled stromal and endothelial cells in corneal homografts. Anat Rec 142:268, 1962
7. Polack FM, Smelser GK: The persistence of isotopically labeled cells in corneal grafts. Soc Exp Biol Med 110:60, 1962
8. Polack FM, Smelser G, Rose J: Long term survival of isotopically labeled stromal and endothelial cells in corneal homografts. Am J Ophthalmol 57:67, 1964
9. Hanna C, Irwin ES: Fate of cells in the corneal graft. Arch Ophthalmol 68:810, 1962
10. Maumenee AE, Kornblueth W: Regeneration of the corneal stromal cells. II. Review of literature and histologic study. Am J Ophthalmol 32:1051, 1949
11. Dunnington JH, Smelser GK: Incorporation of S³⁵ in healing wounds in normal and devitalized corneas. Arch Ophthalmol 60:116, 1958
12. Leblond CP, Nessier B, Kopriwa B: Thymidine-H³ as a tool for the investigation of the renewal of cell populations. Lab Invest 8:296, 1959
13. Basu PK, Miller I, Ormsby HL: Sex chromatin as a biologic cell marker in the study of the fate of corneal transplants. Am J Ophthalmol 49:513, 1960
14. Espiritu RB, Kara GB, Tabowitz D: Studies on the healing of corneal grafts. II. The fate of the endothelial cells of the graft as determined by sex chromatin studies. Am J Ophthalmol 52:91, 1961
15. del Rio Hortega P: El método del carbonato Argentico. Revision general de sus técnicas. Arch Hist Norm Patol 2:165, 1942
16. Dohlman CH: On the fate of the corneal graft. Acta Ophthalmol 35:286, 1957
17. Polack FM, Smelser GK, Rose J: The fate of cells in heterologous corneal transplants. Invest Ophthalmol 4:355, 1963
18. Polack FM: Isotopic labeling of corneal stromal cells prior to transplantation. Transplantation 1:83, 1963
19. Klen R, Hradil I: A contribution to the biology of the corneal graft. Keratoplasty, In Kurz J (ed): Proc Sympos Prague, 1960 Praha, Czechoslavakian Academy of Science, 1962, p 251
20. Brightbill FW, Polack FM, Slappey T, et al: A comparison of two methods for cutting donor corneal buttons. Am J Ophthalmol 75:3, 1973
21. Bourne WM, Kaufman HE: The endothelium of clear corneal transplants. Arch Ophthalmol 94:1730, 1976
22. Carrol JM, Kuwabara T: A classification of limbal epitheliomas. Arch Ophthalmol 73:545, 1965
23. Castroviejo R: Transplantation of cornea, In Peer LA (ed): Transplantation of Tissues. Baltimore, Williams & Wilkins, 1959, pp 137–161
24. Geeraets WJ, Lieb WA, Chan G, et al: Immunochemical analysis of experimental corneal transplants. Am J Ophthalmol 49:740, 1960
25. Maumenee AE, Kornblueth W: Symposium: Corneal transplantation IV. Physiopathology. Am J Ophthalmol 31:1384, 1948
26. Paufique L, Offret G: Étude anatomique et clinique d'une greffe cornéen non perforante. Bull Soc Ophthalmol Fr 60:125, 1947
27. Magitot A: Recherches experimentales sur la survie possible la cornee conservee en de hors de l'organisme et sur la keratoplastie d'huee. Ann Ocul (Paris) 146:1, 1911
28. Babel J: Le sort des greffons corneennes transplantes. Ophthalmologica 109:1, 1945
29. Katzin HM, Kuo PK: Histologic study of experimental corneal transplantation. Am J Ophthalmol 31:171, 1948

30. Arkin W, Czrski P, Trzcinska-Dabrowska Z: Experiments concerning problems of the survival of corneal grafts, *In* Kurz J (ed): Keratoplasty Proc Sympos Prague, 1960. Praha, Czechoslavakian Academy of Science, 1962, p 215

31. Khodadoust AA, Silverstein AM: The survival and rejection of epithelium in experimental corneal transplants. Invest Ophthalmol 8:169, 1969

32. Silverstein AM, Rossman AM, Leon AS: Survival of donor epithelium in experimental corneal homografts. Am J Ophthalmol 69:448, 1970

33. Salceda RS: Endothelial cell survival after keratoplasty in rabbits. Arch Ophthalmol 78:745, 1967

34. Michels R, Kenyon K, Maumenee AE: Retrocorneal fibrous membrane. Invest Ophthalmol 11:822, 1973

35. Harkness RD, Marko AM, Muir HM, et al: The metabolism of collagen and other proteins of the skin of rabbits. J Biochem 56:558, 1954

36. Neuberger A, Slack HGB: The metabolism of collagen from liver, bone, skin, and tendon in the normal rat. J Biochem 53:47, 1953

37. Neuberger A: *In* Brown R, Danielli JF (eds): Metabolism of Collagen Under Normal Conditions. Symposia of the Society for Experimental Biology IX. New York, Academic, 1955, p 72

38. Jackson DS: Chemistry of the fibrous elements of connective tissue, *In* Page IH (ed): Connective Tissue, Thrombosis, and Atherosclerosis. New York, Academic, 1959

39. Smelser GK, Ozanics V: The effect of vascularization on the metabolism of the sulfated mucopolysaccharides and swelling properties of the cornea. Am J Ophthalmol 48:418, 1959

40. Herrmann H, Barry SR: Protein synthesis and tissue integrity in the cornea of the developing chick embryo. Arch Biochem Biophys 55:526, 1955

41. Lowry OH, Gilligan DR, Katersky EM: The determination of collagen and elastin in tissues with results obtained in various normal tissues from different species. J Biol Chem 139:795, 1941

42. Gross J: Studies on the formation of collagen: I. Properties and fractionation of neutral salt extract of normal guinea pig connective tissue. J Exp Med 107:247, 1958

43. Wirtschafter ZT, Bentley JP: The influence of age and growth rate on the extractable collagen of skin of normal rats. Lab Invest 11:316, 1962

44. van Robertson BW: Influence of ascorbic acid on N^{15} incorporation into collagen in vivo. J Biol Chem 197:495, 1952

45. Smelser GK, Polack FM, Ozanics V: Persistence of donor collagen in corneal transplants. Exp Eye Res 4:349, 1965

46. Bostrom H: On the sulfate exchange of sulpho-mucopolysaccharides, *In* Asboe-Hansen G (ed): Connective Tissue in Health and Disease. Copenhagen, Einar Munksgaard, 1954, p 57

47. Bostrom H, Gardell S: Uptake of sulfates in mucopolysaccharides esterified with sulphuric acid in the skin of adult rats after intraperitoneal injection of S^{35}-labeled sodium sulfate. Acta Chem Scand 7:216, 1953

48. Odeblad E, Bostrom H: An autoradiographic study of the incorporation of S^{35}-labeled sodium sulfate in different organs of adult rats and rabbits. Acta Pathol Microbiol Scand (B) 31:339, 1952b

49. Dohlman CH, Bostrom H: Uptake of sulfate by mucopolysaccharides in the rat cornea and sclera. Acta Ophthalmol 33:455, 1955

50. Dohlman CH: Incorporation of radioactive sulfate into the rabbit eye. Acta Ophthalmol 35:115, 1957

51. Dohlman CH: On the metabolism of the corneal graft. Acta Ophthalmol 35:303, 1957

52. Dohlman CH: On the fate of the corneal graft. Acta Ophthalmol 35:20, 1957

Chapter 3

Physiology of the Corneal Graft

The transparency of the cornea is due to its anatomical structure, as well as to its histochemical properties.[1] Any situation in which the anatomical structure of the corneal stroma is altered because of inflammation or physical injury induces the formation of abnormal collagen material or scar tissue, which is usually followed by new vessel growth. In some diseases, loss of transparency is caused by alterations of the corneal epithelium and tear film deficit. The cornea is one of the most exquisitely innervated organs, and denervation often causes epithelial ulceration and loss of transparency. The exact mechanism of epithelial disease due to denervation is not well known, but it is believed that it may be secondary to a reduced blinking rate and uneven tear dispersion. However, corneal grafts that are denervated for several months may retain normal epithelium and normal transparency on the basis of a compensatory increased blinking rate and increased tear production due to the irritation caused by healing and sutures.

Excluding immunologic differences, the structural similarity of host and graft suggest that the metabolic behavior of the latter is the same as that of the surrounding host. In studying the nutritional requirements of the cornea, Maurice[2] estimated that corneal grafts receive adequate amounts of electrolytes, since most of them enter the cornea across the endothelium. He found that oxygen crosses the epithelium or endothelium without resistance and that the O_2 from the atmosphere is the most important. There is minimal oxygen supply from the limbal circulation. Amino acids are present in the anterior chamber in a concentration similar to that in blood plasma. Since they have a molecular size similar to or smaller than fluorescein, experimental studies on the diffusion of this nonmetabolic have shown that most of its penetration into the cornea occurs across the endothelium, and a small proportion is through the limbus. Maurice feels that even in the absence of an active transport mechanism, the supply of amino acids is enough for the nutrition of the corneal graft. The same applies to oxygen and glucose, provided its access to the endothelium is adequate.

The nutritional supply, except for atmospheric oxygen, may not be the same in transplants grafted to vascularized corneas or in eyes with anterior chamber inflammation. Unquestionably, histologic changes in the donor cornea due to handling of the graft at the time of surgery and the process of healing may induce some alterations in the metabolic behavior of corneal transplants, as will be discussed later. The grafted cornea probably behaves as normal corneal tissue in areas distant from the border traumatized by scissors and sutures, where an active process of repair is present. Even though experimental data do not exist, it is assumed that the normal transplant uses atmospheric oxygen for its

metabolism and uses the metabolites diffused from tears and aqueous humor. It is also known that water permeability is increased in corneas with damaged or altered epithelium and endothelium, but the increased permeability will decrease when these two layers are regenerated or the epithelium is replaced with a semipermeable membrane, such as a soft contact lens. The metabolic activity of the endothelium is demonstrated when swollen corneas, which have been kept at 4°C, thin rapidly as soon as its metabolic pump is activated by a rise in temperature. This is called the "temperature reversal effect,"[2-5] which has been well studied to determine the viability of donor corneal tissue.[6,7] The demonstration by Maurice that it is an active endothelial pump that keeps the cornea deturgesced[8] has been subsequently demonstrated by several authors[9-14] in excised corneas, and it points out the importance of this layer in graft transparency. According to Harris,[14] hydration of the cornea depends essentially on the integrity of its layers; water and electrolytes move across the endothelium and evaporate continuously across the epithelium.

Corneal grafts are usually well accepted by the host and enjoy a high rate of success in good prognosis cases (keratoconus, avascular scars, traumatic lesions, etc.). Not long ago, however, the biologic mechanisms that induced graft cloudiness were unknown. The reasons why corneal grafts are usually well accepted and why, in some instances, they become cloudy have been the subject of concern and research by many investigators; from these studies, we have obtained information that allows us to separate the causes of graft failure due to anatomical and physiologic alterations (primary donor failure) to other causes of opacification, such as inflammation, glaucoma, or graft reaction. It is of interest that as far back as 1878, having tried heterologous grafts, Power decided that for a corneal graft to remain clear, it should be homologous tissue. The immunologic picture today is perhaps the most important problem in corneal grafting, particularly in vascularized corneas.

Corneal transplantation follows the same rules that have been laid down for organ transplantation: (1) proper selection and preparation of recipient; (2) donor tissue selection, matching, and careful handling; (3) meticulous surgical techniques, because it is well known that trauma to the donor tissue and poor surgical technique will decrease the success rate of any type of graft; and (4) prevention and control of homograft reaction.

The immediate postoperative period is perhaps the most critical time for a corneal graft from the physiologic point of view. The metabolic demands are great for this tissue that must regenerate its epithelial and endothelial layers, become thinner, and regain transparency while healing occurs at the host–graft junction.

Preservation of the endothelial layer and its protection throughout the surgical procedure is routinely done. The role of the epithelium however, has been ignored until recently, when it was realized that its integrity was preferable to its removal before surgery with the purpose of decreasing its antigenicity. A graft with an intact epithelium and Bowman's layer will have a faster recovery of its transparency. To a great extent, the precorneal tear film also helps the cornea to acquire a normal physiologic state and transparency. According to Mishima and Hedbys,[12] the tear film has a notable influence on the maintenance of corneal hydration and corneal thickness because of changes in fluid tonicity. In addition, white cells and other cellular elements involved in wound healing are

found dispersed in the precorneal film participating in graft healing and adaptation.

Dehydration of a corneal graft, therefore, will occur because of the endothelial pump effect, fluid evaporation, increased tonicity of the tear fluid , and decreased blinking rate.[16] The decreased blinking rate increases tear evaporation and concentration; this hypertonic solution will influence the flow of water in the stroma across the epithelium, and it will become thinner. This is a point to consider in the postoperative management of graft edema, because leaving the eye uncovered may help to treat this condition, as long as the epithelium is intact. It should be remembered that healing of the graft epithelium over the graft–host junction area depends very much on the integrity of the host epithelium and the ability of the recipient eye to produce tear fluid. Defective epithelial healing will be observed in eyes with previous epithelial disease or subepithelial fibrous membranes as well as in dry eyes.

A clear corneal graft should contain about 78% water, which is the proportion found in a normal cornea. Swelling of corneal stroma depends on the amount of water retention by polysaccharides, two-thirds of which are keratan sulfate. It is well known that the swelling effect of the excised cornea is higher than that of the cornea in vivo, and to a great extent, this control of the "in vivo" corneal swelling is effected by the intraocular pressure and a negative imbibition[15] pressure, which seems to be maintained by an active mechanism.[12]

According to Maurice,[2,7,8,18] electrolytes and dissolved substances circulate across the cornea by diffusion, since there is no true flow of water. Particles of the size of human hemoglobin (64 Å) can diffuse easily in corneal stroma, and the same is true for glycogen, which is the main metabolic supply for the cornea.[2] In the cornea, glycogen is found mostly in the epithelium. The total concentration of corneal glycogen is about half of that found in aqueous humor. This amount probably is not large enough to meet the requirements of the cornea, but a certain amount diffuses in from limbal vessels. The center portion of the

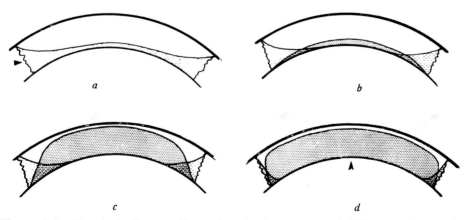

Figure 3-1. Maurice's diagram illustrating the importance of different pathways for corneal nutrition. Albumin and fluorescein or substances of medium-sized molecular weight penetrate the cornea to the limbal stroma (*a* and *b*). Substances of smaller molecular weight (*c* and *d*) reach the corneal stroma through the endothelium, particularly glucose and oxygen. The major source of oxygen, however, is through the corneal epithelium.

cornea, according to Maurice, gets its glucose from the anterior chamber (Fig. 3-1). The nutritional pathways in a recently grafted cornea have important implications, since nutrition for the peripheral portions of a large graft must come across the wound and, for the central portion of the graft, must come through diffusion from the anterior chamber. The pathways may be impaired in situations where the anterior chamber of aphakic eyes and the posterior aspect of the graft is covered with vitreous humor.[17]

In chapter 14, we will discuss the effect of increased intraocular pressure on the corneal graft because of its influence on corneal thickness. It is considered that when the intraocular pressure rises over 40 mm Hg and persists for a long period of time, endothelial damage and corneal edema will occur. However, if the pressure increases rapidly to over 60 mm Hg, water will be pushed out of the stroma with further thinning of the graft.

REFERENCES

1. Payrau P, Pouliquen Y, Faure JP, et al: La Transparence de la Corneé. Paris, Masson et Cie, 1967
2. Maurice DM: Nutritional aspects of corneal grafts and prostheses, *In* Rycroft PV (ed): Corneo-Plastic Surgery, II. International Corneo-Plastic Symposium. London, Pergamon, 1967, p 197
3. Dawson H: The hydration of the cornea. Biochem J 59:24, 1955
4. Harris JE, Nordquist LT: The hydration of the cornea. I. The transport of water from the cornea. Am J Ophthalmol 40:100, 1955
5. Langham ME, Taylor IS: Factors affecting the hydration of the cornea in the excised eye and the living animal. Br J Ophthalmol 40:321, 1956
6. Harris JE: The physiological control of corneal hydration. Am J Ophthalmol 44:262, 1957
7. Hoefle F: Human corneal donor material. Arch Ophthalmol 82:361, 1969
8. Maurice DM: The permeability of sodium ions of the living rabbit cornea. J Physiol 112:367, 1951
9. Brown S, Hedbys BO: The effect of ouabain on the hydration of the cornea. Invest Ophthalmol 4:216, 1965
10. Kaye G, Cole JD, Donn A: Electron microscopy: Sodium localization in normal and ouabain treated transporting cells. Science 150:1167, 1965
11. Hedbys BO, Mishima S: The flow of water in the corneal stroma. Exp Eye Res 4:262, 1962
12. Mishima S, Hedbys BO: The permeability of corneal epithelium and endothelium to water. Exp Eye Res 6:10, 1967
13. Langham ME, Kostelnik M: The effect of ouabain on the hydration and the adenosine triphosphate activity of the cornea. Pharmacol Exp Ther 150:398, 1965
14. Kaye G, Donn LA: Studies on the cornea IV. Some effects of ouabain on pinocytosis and stromal thickness in the rabbit cornea. Invest Ophthalmol 4:844, 1965
15. Harris JE: Current thoughts on the maintenance of corneal hydration in vivo. Arch Ophthalmol 78:126, 1967
16. Mishima S, Maurice DM: The oily layer of the tear film and evaporation from the corneal surface. Exp Eye Res 1:39, 1961
17. Fishbarg J, Stuart J: The effect of vitreous humor on fluid transport by rabbit corneal endothelium. Invest Ophthalmol 14:497, 1975
18. Maurice DM: Anatomia e fisiologia della cornea trapiantata. *In*: Simposio sulla Cheratoplastica. Atti della Soc. Oftal., Milan, Lombarda, 1963, p 97

Chapter 4

The Healing of Corneal Grafts

Even though the scar of the corneal graft is an area less than 2 mm in width, it is one of the most important structures of the grafted cornea, particularly in the immediate postoperative stage and early postoperative period. There is experimental evidence that irregular scars with traumatized graft borders, due to improper cutting and suturing, may affect the graft transparency, influence the development of graft vascularization and rejection, or end in wound dehiscence. Microsurgical techniques and better suture material have improved the results of corneal wound healing; however, it must be remembered that stromal healing depends mostly on keratocytes from the host and the activation of these cells over the wound area.[1-4]

The literature on corneal wound healing is rather extensive and will not be discussed in this chapter. Attention must be brought to the fact that differences in healing may occur in vascular and avascular corneas, as well as in corneas with defective epithelium, subepithelial fibrous membranes, or retrocorneal membranes. In this chapter, the anatomical and functional changes that occur at the host–graft junction during the healing of experimental penetrating allografts will be described.

MATERIALS AND METHODS

The morphology of the scar of the graft was studied by routine histological sections in paraffin-embedded corneas, frozen sections, scanning electron microscopy and transmission electron microscopy.

Participation of Host–Donor Cells and Fibroblastic Activity in the Scar

The participation of host or donor cells in the scar of the graft was studied in tissue labeled with 2 μCi of tritiated thymidine (New England Nuclear Corp., 36 cM/m) by (A) one single injection into the anterior chamber, 24 hr before enucleation at 5, 7, and 14 days after keratoplasty; (B) in donor corneas several weeks prior to surgery;[5] or (C) in corneas where only the recipient (stromal or endothelial cells) had been labeled and autoradiographically studied by a method previously described.[5]

Fibroblastic activity in the scar was studied by determining the amount of ground substance formation (sulfated mucopolysaccharides). Injections of 200 μCi of ^{35}S-labeled sodium sulfate were done in the anterior chamber of 4-wk-old grafts, or 1 mCi/kg intravenously. Contact radioautographs were made following a method previously reported.[6]

Sutures

The effects of sutures on the wound were studied by using two different types of material, 8′ 0′ black silk and 10′ 0′ monofilament nylon. This latter suture was used in a continuous or interrupted form, and the histologic appearance of the wound was evaluated at 7 and 12 days. The study was done in hematoxylin-eosin stained sections or in preparations for the scanning electron microscope. In addition, two experiments were done in collaboration with Drs. R. Eve and R. Troutman, where penetrating grafts were done in rhesus monkeys with interrupted or running monofilament nylon placed at normal depth or through-and-through the cornea.[7]

Scanning Electron Microscopy

Specimens were fixed in 4% glutaraldehyde, rinsed, dehydrated in alcohols of increased gradation, and dried in a critical-point machine (Bomar) or in a freeze-drying apparatus.[8] Samples were coated with gold palladium and examined in a Cambridge Stereoscan microscope at 20 kV. Pictures were recorded on Polaroid P/N film.

Transmission Electron Microscopy

Corneas to be examined by transmission electron microscopy were fixed in 4% osmium tetroxide buffered with 0.15 M sodium cacodylate, pH 7.4, at 4°C. The cornea and the corneal graft were cut into smaller pieces, then the tissue was fixed again for an additional hour and dehydrated through a series of graded alcohols. While in 80% ethanol, the cornea was cut in 1- to 2-mm blocks and embedded in Epon 812 after infiltration with propylene oxide. Thin sections were cut with glass or diamond knives and mounted on toluidine-coated copper meshes, double stained with uranil and lead citrate, and examined in a Siemmens Elmiscope 1.

Experimental Grafts

Penetrating homografts were performed in albino rabbits (3 kg) under aseptic conditions. The animals were anesthetized with sodium pentobarbital (30 mg/kg) and 6- or 6.5-mm grafts were performed. Usually, a pair were operated at the same time and their grafts exchanged. One drop of heparin (10,000 U) was placed in the anterior chamber to reduce the amount of fibrinous aqueous. All surgery was done under an operating microscope. Topical antibiotics and 1% atropine drops were used daily for 1 wk until the sutures were removed or as long as the experiment lasted.

RESULTS

Epithelial Healing

In the rabbit cornea, the morphology of the scar of the graft can be altered by modifying the structure of the host tissue or by using suture material of various kinds. In normal host and graft corneal tissues, cells from both sides will contribute to heal the wound. In recently removed fresh donor corneas, the contribution of host and donor epithelial cells is roughly 50/50. Corneal epithelium heals over penetrating wounds by sliding and by mitosis; it produces a characteristic epithelial plug almost two-thirds deep into the anterior corneal wound with a progressive retraction towards the corneal surface within the first week. It was believed that graft epithelium was replaced 8–12 days after grafting; however, the studies of Khodadoust and Silverstein,[9] by means of immunologic rejections, indicate that most of these cells can persist for long periods of time.

Stromal Healing

The participation of host or donor cells in the scar of the graft, particularly stromal and endothelial cells, was studied in our laboratory by (A) injecting tritiated thymidine into the anterior chamber of recently performed corneal grafts; (B) by grafting corneal tissue with labeled keratocytes or endothelial cells;[5] and (C) by placing nonlabeled corneal transplants in eyes with labeled stromal cells. Our results indicated that when immediate keratoplasties (grafts exchanged between two animals) with tagged host tissue were performed, labeled keratocytes were found in the scar of the wound during the first week after surgery. This same situation developed when the donor tissue had been previously labeled. In this fashion, it was estimated that almost equal numbers of labeled cells appeared in the wound when either one of these two tissues had been labeled. When the isotope was injected into the anterior chamber at 3, 5, or 7 days after keratoplasty, again almost equal numbers of labeled cells were seen at either side of the wound (Figs. 4-1 and 4-2). Initially, these keratocytes transform into fibroblasts and arrange themselves at right angles to the line of incision; however, eventually, they acquire an orientation parallel to the edge of the wound, with many crisscrossing collagen fibers from host to graft. When sutures

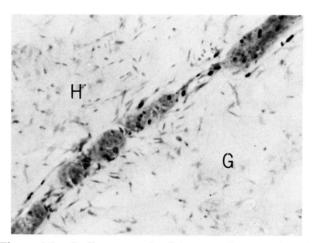

Figure 4-1. Radioautograph of the scar of a corneal graft labeled with tritiated thymidine 24 hr after keratoplasty. In this tangential section, are labeled fibroblasts on either side of the wound, as well as labeled epithelial cells that have insinuated into the wound area (×100; H, host; G, graft).

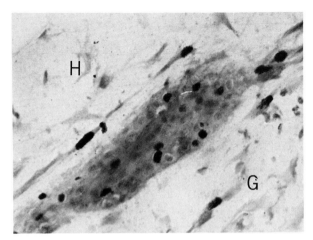

Figure 4-2. This radioautograph, at higher magnification, shows labeled keratocytes on the graft and on the host sides aligned parallel to the corneal wound (×400; H, host; G, graft).

are inserted, fibroblasts will arrange along the suture material and form a scar at right angles to the line of incision (Fig. 4-3). How many host or stromal cells participate in this bridge of fibroblasts induced by suture material is unknown; however, it may be assumed that in this situation, a higher number of host cells may participate when grafts are several hours old.

Between these fibrous bridges, the arrangement of fibroblasts making the scar continues in a circular fashion (Fig. 4-4). The space between the host and the

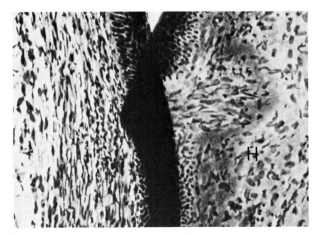

Figure 4-3. Tangential section of a corneal graft showing a circular arrangement of fibroblastic cells along the wound edge. On the host side, fibroblastic cells are arranged in a radial fashion, which corresponds to the location of a corneal suture (Rio-Hortega silver stain; ×200; H, host).

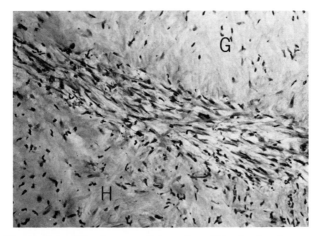

Figure 4-4. The host–graft junction, 2½ wk after kerato-plasty, shows the circular disposition of collagen fibers at the site of the scar. This area corresponds to a portion of the scar between two 8′ 0′ silk sutures (hemotoxylin and eosin; ×200; H, host; G, graft).

graft, which is usually filled by a small amount of fibrin, has been invaded by fibroblastic cells that tend to acquire a circular orientation (Fig. 4-5).

When the midstromal area of the scar was examined with the transmission electron microscope 2 wk after penetrating keratoplasties, elongated cells with prominent endoplasmic reticulum and filamentary condensation in the periph-

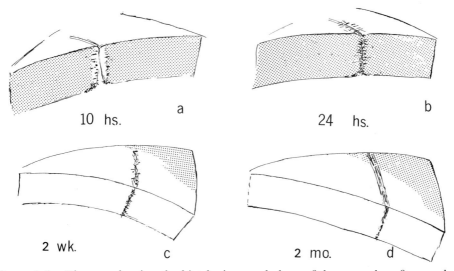

Figure 4-5. Diagram showing the histologic morphology of the corneal graft wound at different times following keratoplasty. **A.** A small area of edge necrosis is repopulated by dividing cells (**B**), which adopt a radial or circular disposition at 24 hr. **C.** Collagen fibrils reach the host–graft junction. **D.** Later they tend to arrange in a circular fashion.

eral cytoplasm were observed. In extracellular spaces, there were small fibrils, which were possible precursors of collagen. Mononuclear and polymorphonuclear leukocytes were frequently seen. In older scars (2–6-mo-old), the area was still very cellular, but mature collagen fibers were present. The most important changes were observed in the deeper corneal layers of the scar, where stromal and Descemet's membrane regeneration had a close relationship. In corneas where the posterior gap was large due to excessive cut of Descemet's membrane in the host and graft, fibrous regeneration was very prominent, and this tissue protruded into the anterior chamber. It is this proliferative connective tissue that originates one type of retrocorneal membrane, as shown by several authors.[10-15]

Incorporation of ^{35}S by Normal and Abnormal Scar Tissue

The incorporation of ^{35}S-labeled sodium sulfate by fibroblasts in the normal scar and at the border of host and graft tissue is shown in Figure 4-6 **A–B**. They correspond to transplants 3–4-wk-old and are characterized by an opaque ring surrounding the graft. The width of this radioactive area is in direct relation to the thickness of the scar in the living eye. In very tight wounds, such as those sutured with continuous nylon material, the scar tends to be rather thin, and there is a narrower ring of ^{35}S incorporation.

The Healing of Descemet's Membrane and Corneal Endothelium

Healing of corneal endothelium follows almost the same pattern as that of corneal epithelium, i.e., by sliding, migration, and mitosis. In studies of tissue labeled with tritiated thymidine, it was observed that the healing of the endothelial border at the host–graft junction showed equal participation of labeled cells on both sides of the wound. Endothelial cells also participate in the formation of the posterior portion of the scar and in the regeneration of Descemet's membrane across the wound. When the posterior edges were in close apposition, a single layer of proliferated and elongated endothelial cells rapidly covered the posterior surface of the scar (Fig. 4-7). The cut edges of Descemet's membrane curled up sharply on the graft side and somewhat less on the host side, perhaps because of the stretching of this layer towards the corneal periphery. When this

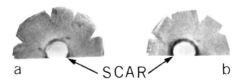

a   SCAR   b

Figure 4-6. Radioautographs of ^{35}S-labeled corneas with transplants 3- and 4-wk-old, respectively. The arrows show increased incorporation of radioactive sulfate by the scar tissue. The amount of density of this scar tissue is less in **A** than in **B**.

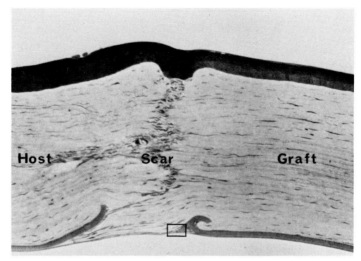

Figure 4-7.   Section of the corneal graft 2 wk after keratoplasty. The posterior cut edges of the host and the graft are in good apposition, and a single layer of endothelial cells lines the scar tissue (×160; reproduced by permission[26]).

area was examined with the electron microscope 2 wk after keratoplasty, the tissue near the cut edges of Descemet's membrane consisted of several layers of elongated cells that could be identified as regenerated endothelial cells (Fig. 4-8). These cells had a large amount of rough surface, endoplasmic reticulum, mitochondria with characteristic longitudinal cristae throughout the cytoplasm, Golgy complex in the perinuclear region, and a terminal web. Many of these cells

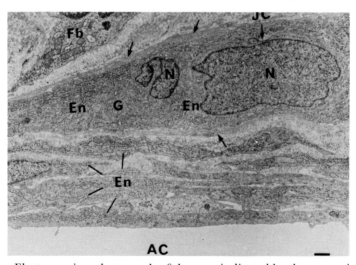

Figure 4-8.   Electron microphotograph of the area indicated by the square in the previous photograph. A multilayer of endothelial cells with prominent endoplasmic reticulum fills the scar tissue. Very thin Descemet's membrane material (arrows) appears between these cells (×6000; EN, endothelial cell; AC, anterior chamber; G, Golgi complex; Fb, fibroblast; N, nucleus; JC, junctionl complex; reproduced by permission.[26])

came in contact with each other, forming junctions, and those closer to the anterior chamber extended small cytoplasmic processes and marginal folds into the anterior chamber. There were elongated endothelial cells within the most posterior portion of the scar, but Descemet's membrane-like material was found around these cells. Spaces between layers of regenerated endothelial cells were filled with fine collagen fibers randomly oriented. In the fibrous tissue between the two edges of Descemet's membrane, there were more mature endothelial cells producing Descemet's membrane material. It appeared that this material was more condensed in areas where endothelial cells were in closer contact with collagen fibers. Those cells that were facing the anterior chamber showed terminal webs. In corneas where the scar was very prominent due to a separation of the two edges of Descemet's membrane, the proliferated fibrous tissue was composed almost entirely of fibroblasts with no evidence of Descemet's membrane deposition. *Two months* following keratoplasty, the posterior wound was fairly well regenerated with a thin Descemet's membrane bridging its two cut edges (Fig. 4-9); however, fibrillar material was interposed between bands of Descemet's membrane material. The posterior surface (anterior chamber) of the scar was covered by a single layer of flat endothelial cells (Fig. 4-10). The new Descemet's membrane at this time measured between 2 and 3 μ, and its ends fused with the curled up borders of Descemet's membrane on the graft and on the host sides. Within the scar, several layers of regenerated endothelial cells were still observed, with Descemet's membrane-like material forming the spaces between each layer of regenerated cells giving the appearance of a multilayer Descemet's membrane. *Six months* after keratoplasty, corneal incisions with poor apposition showed an elongated fibrous mass that appeared as if the cells had been transformed into keratocytes; however, by electron microscopy, many of these cells seemed to be endothelial. These endothelial cells within the scar

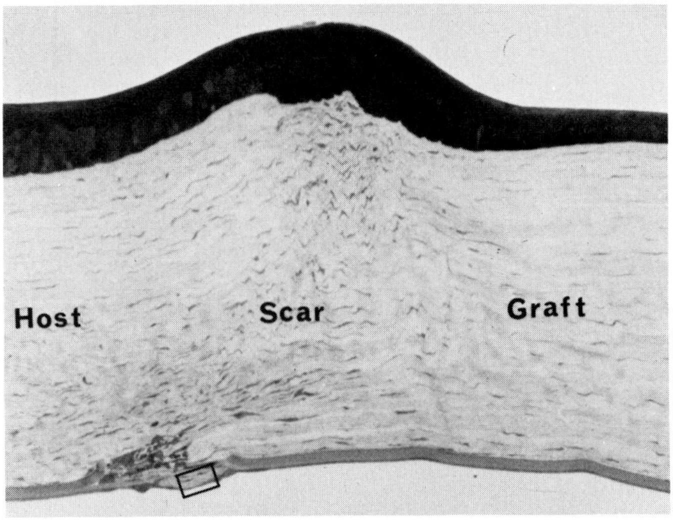

Figure 4-9. Cross-section of a clear graft 2 mo after transplantation. The posterior portion of the scar is in good apposition, and a single layer of endothelial cells bridges the scar tissue (×180; reproduced by permission[26]).

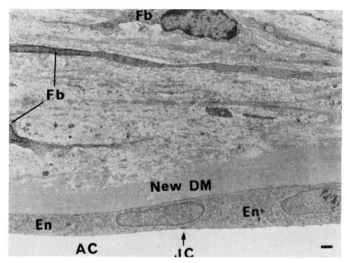

Figure 4-10. Electron micrograph of the area indicated by the square in the previous photograph. The thickness of the new Descemet's membrane in only one-third of the normal Descemet's membrane (×4500; DM, Descemet's membrane; EN, endothelial cell; AC, anterior chamber; Fb, fibroblast; JC, junctional complex. Reproduced by permission[26]).

contain many mitochondria with longitudinal cristae and were surrounded by thin Descemet's membrane material. At this time, the new Descemet's membrane had become thicker, it measured 5–6 μ and was covered by a single layer of normal endothelial cells.

It was frequently found that host endothelial cells labeled with tritiated thymidine had moved towards the graft, regenerating areas of cell destruction in the donor tissue. Whereas this process may occur in the experimental cornea, this type of endothelial cell migration from host to graft has not been documented in the human. The morphology of endothelial cells during the stages of healing of the posterior cornea injury has also been observed with the scanning electron microscope. They actually look like fibroblasts (Fig. 4-11) during the active stage of healing, and when they eventually settle, they round up and acquire the flat appearance of normal endothelial cells. These observations indicate that in rabbit eyes, endothelial cells rapidly proliferate, elongate, and completely cover the posterior surface of the graft scar; within 2 wk, a thin layer of new Descemet's membrane material is produced. Fibroblasts also proliferate within the scar, but they do not protrude into the anterior chamber or disrupt the layer of regenerated endothelium. In cases of poor wound apposition, or when Descemet's membrane has been destroyed because of poor surgical technique, hyperplasia of fibrous tissue forms a mass of spindle-shaped cells and fibers that protrude into the anterior chamber and may give origin to fibrous retrocorneal membranes. Wounds with good apposition show a Descemet's membrane of almost normal thickness at 6 mo, but in cases with fibroblastic overgrowth, no Descemet's membrane material can be found. In experimental situations, Rycroft[11] showed that stromal cells had a tendency to grow in the anterior chamber until limited by a covering of regenerating endothelium. Simi-

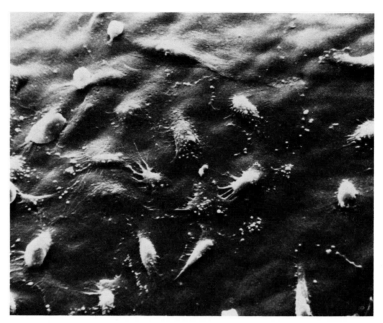

Figure 4-11. Scanning electron microphotograph of fibroblast-looking endothelial cells during the course of wound healing (SEM, ×500).

lar observations were made by Brown and Kitano[12] and were described by Kurz and D'Amico[44] and also by Sherrard.[13] According to Morton et al.,[45] the new Descemet's membrane tends to grow in the rabbit cornea to about 50% of its original thickness in 90 days, and to normal thickness in 1–2 yr following keratoplasty. In our study, an almost normal thickness Descemet's membrane was observed at the end of 6 mo in grafts in which the posterior wound was well approximated. Variations in the cut edges and in the apposition of the posterior host–graft junction influenced the development and formation of new Descemet's membrane. These observations are of importance because, as we will see later, the host–graft junction, devoid of regenerated Descemet's membrane, functions as an open door for lymphocytes and plasma cells to reach the graft endothelium during the rejection process. It is estimated that in the human, Descemet's membrane does not fully regenerate across the host–graft junction for at least 6–9 mo following keratoplasty in situations where the posterior wound apposition is adequate and no iris or vitreous fibrils are incarcerated in the wound.

The Influence of Suture Materials on the Healing of Corneal Grafts

In experimental corneal grafts, it can be observed that the width of the scar (or the space between host and graft) can be almost eliminated by a tight running suture, whether it is silk or nylon. The effect is more pronounced with nylon material, most likely due to the elastic nature of the fiber. Penetrating homokeratoplasties sutured with the above-mentioned materials showed that when nylon material was used in an interrupted fashion, there was an extreme approximation of wound edges with compression of the tissue by the suture. The tissue showed distortion of the corneal fibers with absence of cellular elements in the sutured area at 7 and 12 days (Figs. 4-12–4-15) and few fibroblasts at the host–graft interface, arranged parallel to the wound edges (circular). When a running suture was used, these points of tissue necrosis were more frequent and followed the lines of suture traction (Fig. 4-16). The incorporation of ^{35}S-sulfate by transplants sutured with this material showed a narrow area of sulfate incorporation as compared with silk-sutured wounds.

Grafts sutured with 8' 0' silk usually had sutures inserted farther apart than those of nylon (Fig. 4-17). The spaces between sutures showed a wider interphase filled with fibroblasts arranged mostly parallel to the incision with crisscrossing collagen fibers. There was moderate distortion of the corneal fibers by the suture and no areas of tissue necrosis, unless a tight running silk suture had been used purposely. Fibroblastic and leukocytic reaction was prominent with silk material, particularly on the host side and distal to the knot (Fig. 4-17). Fibroblasts would follow the line of traction of the silk suture and eventually would form a bridge of fibrous tissue between host and graft as previously shown. In the rabbit, the fibrous bridge vascularizes after 2 wk.

It was observed by Eve, in experiments in rhesus monkeys,[7] that if nylon sutures are placed through-and-through the endothelium, a fibrous bridge would develop that would confer great tensile strength to these scars (Fig. 4-18).

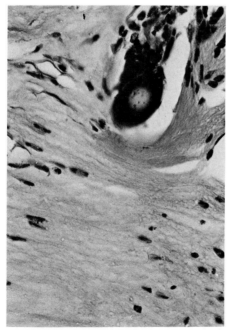

Figure 4-12. Section of host cornea sutured with 10' 0' nylon showing an area absent of stromal cells between the suture and the edge of the graft (hematoxylin and eosin, ×200).

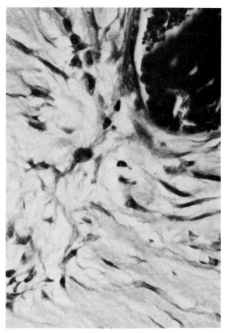

Figure 4-13. A segment of the host stroma sutured with 8'
0 silk, showing alteration of stromal fibers and a decreased
number of corneal cells between the suture and the edge of
the graft (hematoxylin and eosin, ×400).

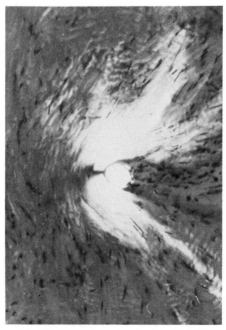

Figure 4-14. Phase-contrast microphotograph of an area
similar to Figure 4-12, showing the distortion of the corneal
collagen fibers induced by the nylon material (×200).

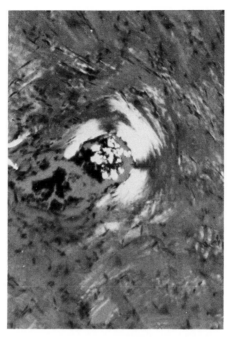

Figure 4-15. Phase-contrast microphotograph of an area of host stroma sutured with 8'0' silk. Disruption of collagen fibers is also evident with this suture but not as pronounced as with the nylon material (×200).

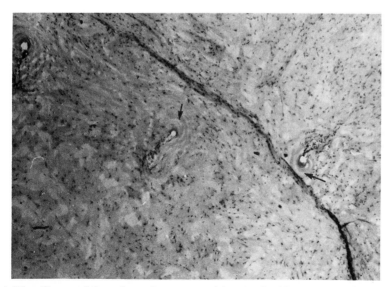

Figure 4-16. Tangential section of a cornea with a 2-wk-old corneal graft sutured with running 10' 0' monofilament nylon. The scar of the graft is thin, but the areas around the monofilament nylon are devoid of fibroblastic cells (arrow) (Hematoxylin and eosin, ×50).

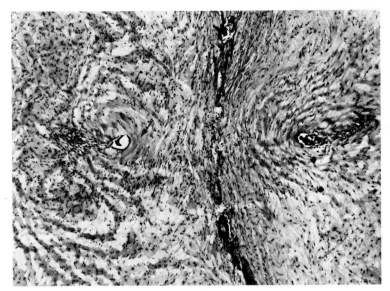

Figure 4-17. Tangential section of a cornea with a 2-wk-old corneal graft sutured with interrupted 8'0' silk. The scar of this graft is more prominent, and even though the area surrounding the suture is relatively devoid of fibroblasts (arrow), a large number of fibroblasts participates in the scar formation (hematoxylin and eosin, ×50).

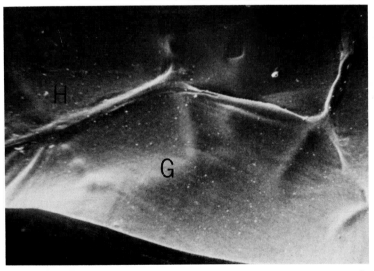

Figure 4-18. Scanning electron microphotograph of an experimental corneal graft with through-and-through sutures, which, two months after keratoplasty, have been covered by endothelial cells (SEM ×50; H, host; G, graft).

Deeply placed nylon sutures, on the other hand, did not prevent wound rupture in grafts of the same age when the cornea was dried prior to examination with the scanning electron microscope.

The Scar as a Pathway for Graft Rejection

It has been shown in earlier studies that sensitized leukocytes can reach the graft endothelium through the scar and across the unhealed Descemet's membrane.[6] These observations have been confirmed in recent studies of experimental graft reactions by means of flat endothelial preparations, transmission and scanning electron microscopy.[15,16] Flat endothelial preparations of the scar tissue at the beginning of the immune reaction show lymphocytes invading the graft endothelium (see chapter 17, Figs. 17-15 and 17-16). These experiments confirm our clinical observations of higher incidence of graft reaction in grafts with wound defects, keratoconus being one of the most common conditions in avascular corneas that shows a high incidence of rejections.[17,28]

COMMENT

Corneal wound healing has been the subject of numerous studies in the past 70 yr.[18] Some earlier studies were concerned with the healing of the graft[19] and the origin of cells forming the scar, particularly those in the anterior and posterior portions of the wound, but as corneal surgery developed, the subject acquired a more practical value. With the advent of fine needles and suture material, the healing of corneal grafts notably improved.

It has been assumed that the scar is a functional and anatomical barrier to cells and vessels from the host,[20] because in opacified grafts, vessels have traversed the scar tissue. However, opaque grafts may also be the result of defective healing, due to faulty tissue apposition, lack of regeneration of Descemet's membrane, and epithelial defects. In regard to epithelial healing over the scar, it is necessary to stress the importance of this type of covering over the wound for adequate healing.[21] In this respect, the use of monofilament nylon in corneal wounds facilitates the growth of epithelium over the suture, since these usually bury into the stroma.

We know from Weimar's studies[22] that corneal cells transform into fibroblasts at the border of the wound during the first 24 hr following surgery; but it is also known[23] that there is a 40–200-μ[24] area of dead keratocytes at the border of the corneal incision, and obviously, this area must be cleaned and repopulated with fibroblasts before reconstruction of the scar is started. Probably the initial perpendicular orientation of keratocytes to the border of the section reflects healing in the edge of the wounded tissue, but once these cells get into the fibrin of the scar itself, they tend to orient themselves along the length of the incision. In very wide scars, such as those obtained experimentally by putting loose sutures, one finds crisscrossing collagen fibers. This cross-over is decreased in scars of tightly sutured wounds, particularly in 10' 0' nylon continuous sutures. We have observed in these studies that multiple interrupted monofilament nylon sutures do not add more strength to the wound but instead decrease it because of necrosis of the wound edge. Silk material can close the wound without being too tightly tied and stimulates enough reaction to form a bridge of fibroblasts between host and graft.

There is a high incidence of wound dehiscence with nylon material as compared to silk (9% versus 2% with silk). This complication is often related to early removal of the suture, but it has also been seen after removing nylon sutures 9 mo after keratoplasty. Reduction of the elasticity of nylon suture or the use of a color indicator in the fiber when excessive tension is applied (D. Willard) are subjects of future research.

Dohlman[25] found increased uptake of ^{35}S at the edge of the wound of penetrating grafts from 8 to 25 days after keratoplasty. The formation of collagen and reticular fibers occurs almost simultaneously with the deposition of ground substance,[1] and both are absent or delayed in devitalized corneas or if epithelium is absent.[21] The increased ^{35}S uptake by thick scars or in grafts with poor apposition has been described previously[25]; ^{35}S was found in abnormal graft wounds in our cases but was decreased in their scars.

In 1964, I proposed that a possible route of graft endothelial cell destruction was the unhealed scar from which immunocompetent cells would gain access to the anterior chamber[6] (Fig. 4-19). Since then, this observation has been confirmed in other experimental and clinical studies.[16,26-29] A gap in the posterior wound of the graft facilitates the development of a weak scar and leaves a door open for endothelial cell destruction in the event of an immune reaction, iris or vitreous adhesions, or the development of retrograft membranes.[27] To eliminate this potential problem, through-and-through suturing of the cornea has been proposed and realized experimentally with 10' 0' monofilament nylon.[7,29] Experimental results are encouraging; however, clinical experience is not available at this time.

The Effect of Corticosteroids and Immunosuppressive Drugs on Corneal Wound Healing

It is well known that topical and systemic corticosteroid administration delays corneal wound healing.[30-39] In penetrating corneal wounds, the number of fibroblasts at the wound edge is usually considered a reliable guideline of scar formation, even though other factors may intervene in the healing process as mentioned previously. Since the fibroblast is the most important element in the production of scar tissue, its behavior in healing injuries in avascular connective tissue, such as the cornea, is most interesting; particularly if one can evaluate the effect of steroids or immunosuppressive drugs on cell function. Stromal healing may occur by migration of fibroblasts from the limbal area, transformation of keratocytes near the wound edges, and mitosis of existing connective tissue cells around the wound, as well as blood-borne connective tissue cells rich in the wound from the surface with the lacrimal tear fluid. One way to determine the activity of scar tissue in the transplanted cornea is by studying the amount of ground substance elaborated by the fibroblasts as detected by the technique of radioactive sulfate incorporation as previously described. Another way is to determine the number of cells undergoing mitosis in the healing area. Since steroids inhibit the proliferation of connective tissue cells, the technique of isotopic DNA labeling would allow a quantitative or a morphologic determination of wound healing activity and DNA inhibition by the application of topical steroids.

The previously described technique of DNA labeling with tritiated thymidine was used in these experiments to determine the effect of topical steroids on wound healing. In order to eliminate the participation of surface epithelial cells as well as blood-borne cells present in the tear film, a nonpenetrating corneal injury was done by freezing the central cornea of rabbits with a cryocautery (−79°C), a technique that has been previously used to label corneal tissue prior to transplantation with the purpose of studying the survival of corneal cells. The round-tipped cryocautery that caused a circular injury was 6 mm in diameter. Two experiments were done.[40] In the first experiment, the number of labeled cells in control corneas were compared to the number of labeled cells in corneas that had been treated with topical steroids (Dexamethasone ointment, 0.05% and Medrysone® suspension, 1%). In the second experiment, the area of the injured cornea was measured in the control and in the treated groups after 5 days of treatment.

In the first experiment, the topical steroids were given to the animals beginning 16 hr after freezing, 3 times a day. Control eyes used saline drops or an antibiotic ointment. Twenty-two hours after the freezing injury (when DNA synthesis usually starts), 2 μCi of tritiated thymidine in 0.1 cc of Eagle's basal media was injected into the anterior chamber of all eyes after evacuation of 2–3 drops of aqueous humor with a 27-gauge needle. This injection was followed by another application of steroid preparation. Twenty-four hours after freezing (2 hr after last steroid application), the animals were killed, the eyes removed and fixed in 10% formalin. The corneas were also removed and prepared for autoradiography. The number of labeled cells were counted and averaged in a series of sections obtained from each cornea.

In the second experiment, corneas were treated with topical steroids, 3 times a day, starting 16 hr after freezing. At 22 hr postfreezing, the corneas were labeled as in the first experiment, but these eyes received topical steroids for 4 additional days. On the fifth day, the eyes were removed 2 hr after the last application of cortisone and fixed in formalin. The corneas were then processed for radioautography as in experiment one.

In the first experiment, autoradiographs of control and cortisone-treated corneas showed incorporation of tritiated thymidine (injected 22 hr after freezing) into a band of cells surrounding the acellular wounded area. The width of the band varied from 2 to 5 to 6 layers of labeled cells, and the size of the ring of labeled cells corresponded roughly to the 6-mm frozen area. The average (mean) number of cells that incorporated the isotope used as controls was 327 cells per section. No significant difference was observed between eyes treated with saline or those treated with the antibiotic ointment; however, the mean number of labeled cells in eyes treated with the steroids was 90 per section, indicating a 73% reduction in the number of cells incorporating the isotope (Fig. 4-19). If the cornea had been treated before and after freezing with the steroids, the uptake of the isotope was further reduced to 59 cells per section, indicating an 82% inhibition of DNA synthesis. At the 24-hr stage, the diameter of the injured area was similar in the steroid-treated group as in the controls. However,

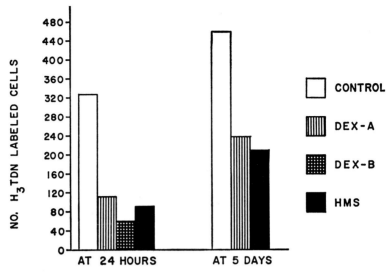

Figure 4-19.   Twenty-four hours following a freezing injury of the cornea, an average of 320 tritium-labeled cells were found around the injured area. The number of labeled cells was reduced in corneas treated with three different types of steroids. Five days later, the number of labeled cells in control corneas, as well as in steroid-treated corneas had increased; however, steroid-treated corneas showed over 70% reduction of labeling.

this difference was very prominent 4 days later. In experiment two (Fig. 4-20), the difference in the healed area between the control and the steroid-treated area was close to 50% (46% for the Medrysone-treated corneas, and 53% for the Dexamethasone-treated corneas). In this experiment, the initial isotopic labeling outlined the size of the injured area at day 1. The number of labeled cells was also different in these two groups of corneas.

These experiments confirm studies by others who reported delayed corneal wound healing after local or systemic use of corticosteroids. They also show that the incorporation of tritiated thymidine by regenerating keratocytes can be inhibited by the topical application of weak steroid medications, such as the 0.05% Dexamethasone ointment used 3 times a day. In other experiments,[41] in which azathioprine (Imuran) was used in similar type of nonperforating injuries as well as in penetrating injuries, we found that the reduction of DNA synthesis and the reduction of tensile strength was about 50% in the injured areas. Whereas the effect appears to be similar, the mechanism of DNA inhibition by topical steroids and immunosuppressive drugs may not be the same. Chemical determination of the amount of DNA present after treatment with steroids should clarify the question of whether these preparations had actually inhibited DNA synthesis, because it is possible that steroids may interfere with cellular production by altering the cell membrane, the ribosomes, or the nucleus. In many of the sections of treated corneas we examined, there were labeled cells in the injured areas, indicating that DNA synthesis had been only partially blocked by the steroids, or the steroid was not available to these cells in enough concentration to start a full inhibitory effect, or perhaps because the mechanism of inhibition was effective only during some stages of DNA synthesis. The effect of steroids seems to be proportional to frequency of application and may be cumulative, because

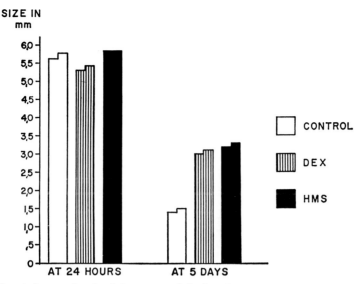

Figure 4-20. A 6-mm circular injury was of similar size at 24 hr. However, 5 days later, the healing area in control corneas was less than 2 mm, while the steroid-treated corneas was twice as large.

Dexamethasone ointment applied for 2 days prior to the injury had greater inhibitory effect on the incorporation of the isotope.

The delay in wound healing seen at the end of 5 days agrees with studies showing decreased tensile strength[38,39] in corneal wounds treated with steroids or by the decrease in the number of fibroblasts,[30-39] although in many of these experiments, the amount of steroid used was greater than the clinical dose. In our experiments,[40] it was obvious that at the end of 5 days, the size (diameter of the injured area) was larger in the steroid-treated corneas as compared to the controls, indicating that there was a good relationship to the decrease in DNA synthesis.

In another series of experiments,[41,42] we studied the effect of 5-iodo-2-deoxyuridine (IDU) on stromal wound healing. These studies were done because in clinical practice, we often treat recent corneal transplants for herpetic keratitis with this antiviral drug. It was important, therefore, to determine if the frequent use of IDU had any deleterious effect upon graft healing. A method of investigation similar to that performed with topical steroids was used. A situation was created whereby a corneal injury was produced by freezing, thus avoiding the participation of surface or anterior chamber macrophages in wound healing. The corneas of adult rabbits were frozen with a round cryoprobe tip producing a 6-mm circular injury. In one experiment, corneas were treated with IDU, 0.1% solution, every 2 hr for 6 hr. Twenty-three hours after freezing, 2μCi of tritiated thymidine were injected into the anterior chamber, and the animals were killed 2 hr later. Controls received saline drops with the same frequency and were labeled at the same period of time. The corneas were fixed in formalin and prepared for radioautographic study as in previous experiments. The number of labeled cells were counted and averaged.

In a second experiment, the frozen corneas were labeled 23 hr after freezing, and experimental corneas were treated with IDU ointment 3 times a day, (every 2 hr), for a period of 5 days. The control corneas received only saline drops. At the end of 5 days, the animals were killed, the eyes removed, and the corneas prepared for radioautography. In this second experiment, the diameter of the unhealed area was measured and compared to the diameter of the unhealed cornea in the control group. The first experiment indicated a 50% reduction of labeled cells in IDU-treated eyes, and in experiment two, the area of unhealed (area devoid of cells) stroma was 50% larger than that of control corneas.

These experiments demonstrated that IDU used in therapeutic doses competes with tritiated thymidine for incorporation into DNA of regenerating keratocytes and that the delay in healing or cell repopulation of the frozen area seems to be related to this inhibition in cell mitosis. These observations seem to be in accordance with experiments of Payrau and Dohlman,[43] who found that the tensile strength of penetrating corneal wounds decreased about 50% in corneas similarly treated with IDU. Since this drug acts by blocking the synthesis of DNA, it should have no effect on the migration of keratocytes from the periphery into the wound and the elaboration of connective tissue. Possibly, this population of migrating keratocytes accounts for the 50% of wound healing observed in Payrau and Dohlman's and in our experiments. The implication of these experiments in relation to penetrating keratoplasties is that when steroids and/or IDU are used during the early stages of wound healing, one must be aware of the reduction in wound strength, so sutures can be left longer and wound dehiscences or ruptures can be prevented.

Biochemical Aspects of Wound Healing

Up to this point, we have discussed the morphologic aspects of corneal wound healing, but little has been said about the biochemical mechanism of stromal healing. We have seen previously that in the absence of epithelium, stromal wounds do not heal.[1,2,4] However, once the process starts, it follows the same type of repair we see in other connective tissues. The knowledge of these mechanisms, even if superficial, is valuable when we realize that we can decrease our demands for repair if we minimize trauma in the host and in the graft. For example, we must remember that an incision in the cornea with a razor blade causes destruction of cells and causes tissue necrosis up to 1 mm of the cut edge.[23] For repair to occur, the damaged stroma must be enzymatically removed,[24] at least partially, by leukocytes that appear in the wound shortly after the injury. Their action and that of macrophages, cause an increase in lactate ions, a pH elevation, and a high PCO_2 gradient in the wound area. Possibly, this gradient stimulates the migration of fibroblasts by releasing chemotactic substances, or it may transform keratocytes into fibroblasts.[3] Vitamin A favors the migration of macrophages into the wound and reverses the inhibition effect of steroids on these cells. Keratocytes transformed to fibroblasts, transformed monocytes, or migrated fibroblasts all converge to the wound to deposit ground substance (proteoglycans or mucopolysaccharides) and collagen (Fig. 4-21). The population of new fibroblasts is controlled by their so called "contact inhibition" and also by the biochemical modification of the wound, which goes along with a reduction in the collagenolytic activity of leukocytes.

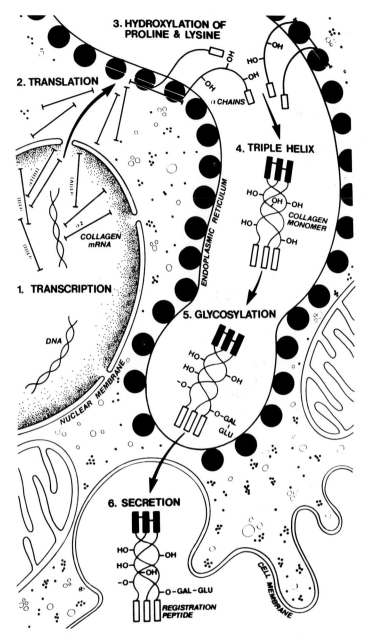

Figure 4-21. Illustration depicting the mechanism of collagen production by a fibroblast. The triple-chain collagen is secreted by the endoplasmic reticulum. Ground substance (mucopolysaccharides) may be produced at the same time. (Reproduced by permission.[48])

At first, newly deposited collagen is almost a gel or tropocollagen (type III collagen, like that found in embryonic tissue; Fig. 4-22). This early collagen is broken down by a collagenase (procollagen peptidase), while more mature collagen is made (type I collagen found in dermis). These two types of collagen differ mostly in the amino acid composition of their alpha-chain (Fig. 4-23).[47] The synthesis of collagen requires the presence of specific amino acids and cofactors, one of the most important being vitamin C. If this vitamin is absent, enzymes that activate the formation of collagen will not work, and the wound will not heal. Steroids also interfere with the fibroblast metabolism in collagen synthesis. Proteoglycans are very large molecules (4000 Å), rich in sulfate and glucoronic groups. They fill spaces between alpha-chains, influencing its linkage and fiber orientation. The two main glycosaminoglycans found in skin and corneal scars

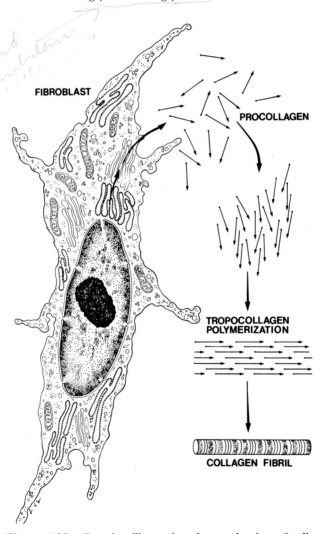

Figure 4-22. Drawing illustrating the production of collagen by a fibroblast and its organization into a mature collagen fibril. (Reproduced by permission.[48])

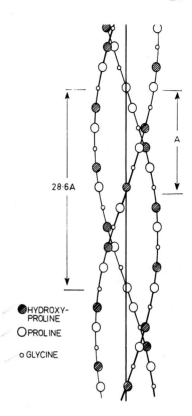

28·6A

●HYDROXY-
PROLINE

○PROLINE

○ GLYCINE

Figure 4-23. Diagram illustrating the triple helix organization of collagen and the sequential distribution of amino acids. (Reproduced by permission.[47])

are chondroitin sulfate and dermatan sulfate, while the main proteoglycan in normal cornea is keratan sulfate. One of the characteristics of these substances is their ability to bind water. As healing progresses, new collagen replaces that removed enzymatically. Collagen fibrils follow lines of stress and the same seems to be true for the proteoglycan molecules, the role of which is not too well defined. Collagen (triple helical) is resistant to proteolytic enzyme destruction, but heat (as low as 39°C) can denature (separate the triple coil) collagen and make it susceptible to digestion by such enzymes. With collagen maturation, the production of proteoglycans decreases, the water they retain is also decreased, and the scar takes on a white appearance.[48]

REFERENCES

1. Dunnington JH, Weimar V: Influence of the epithelium on the healing of corneal incisions. Am J Ophthalmol 45:89, 1958
2. Dunnington JH, Smelser GK: Incorporation of S[35] in healing wounds in normal and devitalized corneas, Arch Ophthalmol 60:116, 1958
3. Weimar V: The sources of fibroblasts in corneal wound repair. Arch Ophthalmol 60:93, 1958
4. Dohlman CH, Gasset AR: Studies on corneal wound healing. Procedures of the Second Corneal Plastic Conference, Pergamon, London, 1967

5. Polack FM, Smelser CK, Rose J: Long-term survival of isotopically labelled stromal and endothelial cells in corneal homografts. Am J Ophthalmol 57:67, 1964

6. Polack FM: Histopathological and histochemical alterations in the early stages of corneal graft rejection. J Exp Med 116:709, 1962

7. Sanchez J, Polack FM, Eve R, et al: Microsurgical sutures II: Endothelial healing in through and through sutures. Can J Ophthalmol 9:42, 1974

8. Polack FM: Scanning electron microscopy of corneal graft rejection: Epithelial rejection, endothelial rejection, and formation of posterior graft membranes. Invest Ophthalmol 11:1, 1972

9. Khodadoust AA, Silverstein AM: The survival and rejection of epithelium in experimental corneal grafts. Invest Ophthalmol 8:169, 1969

10. Hales RH, Spencer WH: Unsuccessful penetrating keratoplasties. Correlation of clinical and histological findings. Arch Ophthalmol 70:805, 1963

11. Rycroft PV: Corneal graft membranes. Trans Ophthalmol Soc UK 85:317, 1965

12. Brown SI, Kitano S: Pathogenesis of the retrocorneal membrane. Arch Ophthalmol 75:518, 1966

13. Sherrard ES, Rycroft PV: Retrocorneal membranes I. Their origin and structure. Br J Ophthalmol 51:379, 1967

14. Sherrard ES, Rycroft PV: Retrocorneal membranes II. Factors influencing their growth. Br J Ophthalmol 51:387, 1967

15. Inomata H, Smelser GK, Polack FM: Fine structure of regenerating endothelium and Descemet's membrane in normal and rejecting corneal grafts. Am J Ophthalmol 70:48, 1970

16. Polack FM: Scanning electron microscopy of the host–graft junction in corneal graft reaction. Am J Ophthalmol 73:704, 1972

17. Chandler J, Kaufman HE: Graft reaction after keratoplasty for keratoconus. Am J Ophthalmol 77:543, 1974

18. Paufique L, Sourdille GP, Offret G: Les Greffes de la Corneé. Paris, Masson et Cie, 1948

19. Castroviejo R: Keratoplasty-microscopic study of the corneal grafts. Trans Am Ophthalmol Soc 35:355, 1937

20. Duke-Elder S: The problems of homoplastic grafting as applied to the cornea. J R Coll Surg Edinb 1:187, 1955

21. Smelser GK: The importance of the epithelium in the synthesis of the sulfated ground substance in corneal connective tissue. Trans NY Acad Sci 21:575, 1959

22. Weimar V: The transformation of corneal stromal cells to fibroblasts in corneal wound healing. Am J Ophthalmol 44:173, 1957

23. Matsuda H, Smelser GK: Electron microscopy of corneal wound healing. Exp Eye Res 16:427, 1973

24. Graf B, Pouliquen Y, Frouin M, et al: The phenomena of reabsorption in the course of cicatrization of experimental wounds of the cornea. Exp Eye Res 13:24, 1971

25. Dohlman CH: On the metabolism of the corneal graft. Acta Ophthalmol (Kbh) 35:303, 1957

26. Inomata H, Polack FM, Smelser CK: Fine structural changes in the corneal endothelium during graft rejection. Am J Ophthalmol 70:48, 1970

27. Polack FM: Corneal graft rejection: Clinico-pathological correlation, In Porter R and Knight J (eds): Corneal Graft Failure, A CIBA Foundation Symposium. London, 1973, pp 127–139

28. Offret G, Pouliquen Y: Les Homogreffes de la Corneé. Societé Francaise d'Ophthalmologie. Paris, Masson, 1974

29. Massey J, Hanna C: Penetrating keratoplasty with the use of through and through nylon sutures. Arch Ophthalmol 91:381, 1974

30. Duke-Elder S, Ashton N: Action of cortisone on tissue reactions of inflammation and repair with special reference to the eye. Br J Ophthalmol 35:695, 1951

31. Ashton N, Cook C: Effect of cortisone on corneal wounds. Br J Ophthalmol 35:708, 1951

32. Rossi A: Prednisone e ferite corneali. Rass Ital d'Ottal 24:430, 1955

33. Leopold IH, Purnell JE, Cannon EJ: Local and systemic cortisone in ocular disease. Am J Ophthalmol 34:361, 1951

34. Gordon DM, McLean, JM, Koteen H, et al: The uses of ACTH and cortisone in ophthalmology. Am J Ophthalmol 34:1675, 1951

35. Newell FW, Dixon JM: The effect of subconjunctival cortisone upon the immediate union of experimental corneal grafts. Am J Ophthalmol 34:977, 1951

36. Palmerton ES: The effect of local cortisone on wound healing in rabbit corneas. Am J Ophthalmol 40:344, 1955

37. McDonald PR, Leopold IH, Vogel AW, et al: Hydrocortisone (Compound F) in ophthalmology: Clinical and experimental studies. Arch Ophthalmol 49:400, 1953

38. Yasuna JM, Ojers GW, Frayer WC, et al: An experimental study of the effect of cortisone on the eye. Am J Ophthalmol 37:923, 1954

39. Aquavella JV, Gasset A, Dohlman CH: Corticosteroids in corneal wound healing. Am J Ophthalmol 58:621, 1964

40. Polack FM, Rosen P: Topical steroids and tritiated thymidine uptake. Arch Ophthalmol 77:400, 1967

41. Polack FM, Rosen P: The effect of cortisone and azathioprine in corneal wound healing. Invest Ophthalmol 5:530, 1966

42. Polack FM, Rose J: The effect of 5-iodo-deoxyuridine (IDU) in corneal wound healing. Arch Ophthalmol 71:520, 1964

43. Payrau P, Dohlman CH: IDU in corneal wound healing. Am J Ophthalmol 57:999, 1964

44. Kurz GH, D'Amico R: Histopathology of corneal graft failures. Am J Ophthalmol 6:184, 1968

45. Morton PL, Ormsby HL, Basu PK: Healing of the endothelium and Descemet's membrane of rabbit corneas. Am J Ophthalmol 46:2, 1958

46. Polack FM: The corneal host–graft junction. Physiopathology of the scar. Arch Ophthalmol (Paris) 35:139, 1975

47. Hall DA: International Review of Connective Tissue Research, vol 1. New York, Academic, 1963

48. Hunt TK, Van Winkle W: Fundamentals of wound management in surgery, wound healing, wound repair. South Plainfield, NJ, Chirurgecom Publ, Smith Kline and French Labs, 1976

Chapter 5

Tissue Transplantation and Histocompatibility

At the beginning of this century, investigators observed that tissue grafts between animals of the same species were destroyed shortly after transplantation. In 1906, Ehrlich[1] proposed that this was due to lack of substances essential for their survival, but his theory was abandoned when it was learned that tissues could be cultivated in vitro in very basic media consisting of saline solutions and homologous or heterologous serum. It was also believed at that time that there was an innate resistance to homologous grafts and that blood-type incompatibility was the main reason for graft intolerance.

According to Batchelor,[2] the earliest experiments on tissue compatibility were genetic rather than serologic. He mentioned that in 1909, Loeb[3] demonstrated that mammary carcinoma obtained from one strain of Japanese mice grew faster if further transplanted to other mice of the same stock; however, mice from other stocks were not susceptible to this tumor. Loeb found that the first generation (F_1) of these two stocks was also susceptible to the tumor; but the F_2 generation produced mice resistant to the tumor. Little,[4] in 1914, explained this problem, indicating that a series of genetic factors existed in these mice that would make them accept the tumor; but, if many of these factors were absent, as it probably occurred in the F_2 generations, the animals would be resistant to the tumor. These genetic principles have been confirmed and apply to normal tissue transplantation. In 1948, Snell[5] suggested that the genes that determine the fate of transplants should be termed "histocompatibility" or "H" genes. Since then, inbreeding of mice has been carried out for genetic and transplantation studies, and today our knowledge of the H-system is greater for these species than for any other. At present, 13 loci have been identified. Eleven are designated by number H-1 through H-11, and the remaining two are referred to as the Y-linked and X-linked systems, since they are related to the sex chromosomes. In mice, the H-2 locus is the most important in determining compatibility of tumor and skin grafts, and this seems to be true also for man.[2] In the human, the analogous transplantation antigens occupy a large portion of the sixth chromosome (HL). They are prominent in most nucleated cells, particularly in epithelial cells and cells from the lymphoid tissue, which is one of the reasons why, in man, the latter are used for tissue typing (HLA or human-leukocyte–locus A).

Woodruff and Allan had already shown in 1953[6] that skin homografts would be destroyed, even if donor and host shared the same red cell antigens known at that time. Since critical matching of human red cell groups between donor and recipient did not prevent the rejection of transplants, it was assumed that human red cells carried only minor or weak H-antigens. However, tissue typing is also done for ABO systems, because man can develop strong sensitization to A and B antigens of bacterial origin, which some believe can influence homograft reactions. ABO typing was also studied in the field of ophthalmology experimentally[7,8] and clinically.[9-11] At present, the feeling is that there is no correlation between blood groups and successful corneal grafts. It should be remembered that ABO compatibility is one of the requirements to avoid immune reactions,[9] and since white cells contain all the HLA antigens, a host can be sensitized with these cells when receiving blood and develop an accelerated graft rejection. The same is true with skin, which shares many antigens with the corneas. Corneal graft rejection after skin grafts has been amply studied experimentally.[12]

In general, most of the earliest studies on tissue transplantation and a large amount of our basic knowledge in this field was done with skin grafts. In the past 15 yr, most important advances of organ transplantation have been not with skin but with kidney and heart. These results, however, cannot match the high rate of successful corneal or cartilage grafts. It is evident that, even though we can perform successful grafts because we have the technology to do it, we have not been able to solve the immune problem, this being more severe in richly vascularized organs. For many years it has been assumed that the success of corneal and cartilage grafts was due not only to the fact that they had few cells and little antigenic material present in the cornea, but also because they could not induce sensitization when placed in an avascular host. It was later proven that the cornea did not have to be placed in a vascularized bed to sensitize a host, since rejections also occurred in avascular corneas.[13] It has also been learned that these tissues have enough cellular material to induce sensitization and that donor cells do not have to die to release antigens. Recent concepts on the ultrastructure and molecular configuration of cell membranes[14] indicate that antigens (polypeptide chains 30,000/11,800 mol wt) are elaborated by the cell and deposited on its outer cell membrane by a process of active molecular transport through membrane pores (Fig. 5-1). These antigens can be released and again be reformed within a few hours,[15,16] thus having a true turnover. This is far from the concept of several years ago, when it was believed that antigens were contained inside the cell and released only after cell death. According to the receptivity of the host, a very small amount of antigenic material is enough to sensitize him and develop a state of immunity that may cause the rapid destruction of a second graft with similar antigenic structure. This phenomenon of the "second set," originally described by Medawar in 1945[17] in studies with skin grafts, laid down the basis for our modern concepts in transplantation. Medawar pointed out that the second set of transplants had been done in sites distant from the original grafts and concluded that the resistance to homografts depended on a systemic rather than a local reaction, indicating development of immunity in the host (acquired immunity). Initially, the concept of immunity meant an inflammatory cellular reaction by host cells around the graft. After Medawar, the acquired immunity hypothesis meant that homotransplants or allografts acted as antigens and evoked the production of cell-bound or circulating antibodies. The second set phenomenon is important because of the presence of similar antigens in various tissues or organs. Infrequently, however, second sets from different donors may

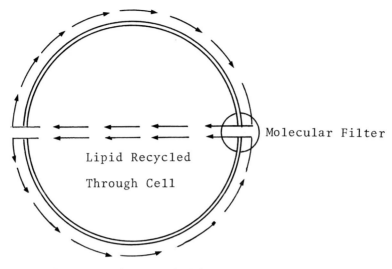

Plasma Membrane Lipid Flow

Figure 5-1. Bretscher schema of a cell, showing the flow of lipid molecules along the cell surface to enter the cell body again through a molecular filter. In this manner, antigens are continuously regenerating, although a number of them are released to the host's lymphatic circulation.

also induce faster graft rejection.[18] Dempster, in 1963,[19] found a faster rate of kidney failure in animals that had previously received grafts. This phenomenon has occasionally occurred with corneal grafts. It has been observed that transplantation of second sets of dissimilar tissues from the same donor may accelerate the destruction of this graft.[20–23] Simonsen et al.[24] found that dogs that had received a whole spleen homograft, or free skin grafts, reacted more violently to a kidney transplant from the same donor than to one of another donor. In 1956, Hardin[25] found an accelerated rate of lung rejection or skin rejection when one of these grafts had been previously performed in dogs. Maumenee[12] found that the transplantation of skin to the subcutaneous area of the abdomen of rabbits with previous corneal grafts induced the rejection of the corneal graft, and similar results were obtained by grafting lymphoid cells.[26,27] All these experiments document the fact that tissues and organs share certain numbers of antigens.

HLA HISTOCOMPATIBILITY SYSTEMS

Major histocompatibility (HL) antigens, as other cellular antigens, are present in the surface of nucleated cells, and their presence is determined by two pairs of genes located in a single large region of the sixth chromosome, (Fig. 5-2).[28,29] The region where these genes are present is now well defined, but new alleles (other genes at the same locus) are being discovered, and the role of the newly described "locus C" is gradually being defined. This whole chromosomal region affects allograft survival as well as immune response and response to certain diseases. The first histocompatibility locus has been called LA (leukocyte

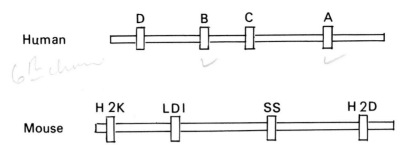

Figure 5-2. Schema of chromosome no. 6, indicating the relative position of male histocompatibility locus in a human and the counterpart in the mouse. A and B locus in the human are the most important histocompatibility antigens at the present time; however, the function of locus C is being defined.

antigen), was formerly called segregant A, and is now renamed HLA-A. The second locus, now called HLA-B, was formerly called second series, series S, or locus Four. Table 5-1 lists the most frequent transplantation antigens.

Since normal individuals have two chromosomes, no. 6, each containing HLA zones A and B, their phenotype consists of two antigens from series A and two from series B. When typing donor tissue, one tries to match these four antigens, and if this happens, then the term "full house" is applied. However, since there are many antigens in each series, it is unlikely to find the same antigens in both donor and host tissues. It has been observed that HLA-A anti-

Table 5-1

Most Frequent Antigens of the HLA System

Locus A (First Series)	Locus B (Second Series)
A1	B5
A2	B7
A3	B8
A9	B12
A10	B13
A11	B14
A12	B17
A28	
A29	B27
AW23	BW15
AW24	BW16
AW25	BW17
AW26	BW21
AW30	BW22
AW31	BW35
AW32	BW37
AW33, etc.	BW38
	BW39
	BW40, etc.

Also, six alleles have been recognized for the incompletely characterized C locus.[30,31]

gens frequently show close reactions between them, and the same is true for HLA-B antigens, but there is no close reactivity with the opposite series. Therefore, it is accepted that if two individuals react with several HLA antigens, it does not mean that they have exactly the same series of antigens, but that the antigens may be showing cross-reactivity. According to Gibbs et al.,[23] individuals classified as HLA serologically identical, may in fact be similar but not identical.

In the Gibbs study, they found that in 100 corneal transplants, more than one-third did not share any antigens, 38% shared one antigen, and 23% shared two antigens. They further observed that whether the recipients shared antigens or not, graft rejections appeared. They were present in about one-fourth of the cases that shared two antigens. It seemed that those grafts that shared no antigens and rejected had irreversible rejections. Also, those with more pronounced host vascularization had a higher incidence of reactions and worse prognosis (Fig. 5-3).

HLA antigens, first described in the cornea by Ehlers and Ahrons[9] and by Stark et al.,[32] document the fact that these antigens exist in all nucleated cells. The alleged decrease in antigenicity of corneas treated by soaking in tissue culture solutions or sera may be due to a noticeable loss of viable cells rather than to a modification of their antigenicity.[20] Allansmith et al.,[33] in a study of 43 nonselected grafts, found that matching for two or four antigens did not correlate with clinical results. However, in Vannas' experience,[34] matching for four antigens improved the results. Possibly a combination of HLA matching with tissue treatment with blocking antiserum[37,38] may improve results of grafts in eyes with poor prognosis.

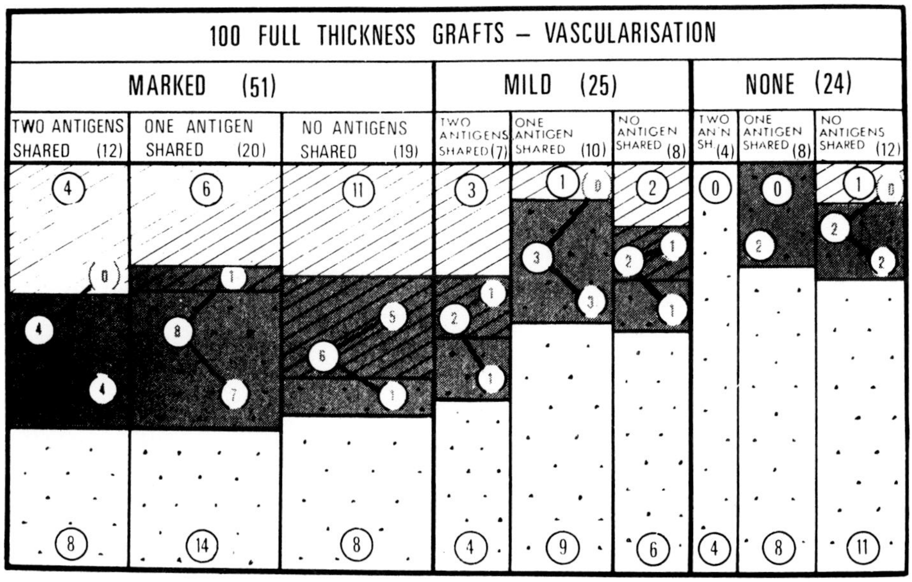

Figure 5-3. Effect of the number of shared antigens and degree of corneal vascularization on the clinical outcome of grafting. Dotted areas correspond to clear grafts. In general, results seem to improve when more antigen is shared. (Shaded area, rejectors; cross-hatched area, cloudy grafts; reproduced by permission.)[23]

In regards to the relation of donor tissue originating from different ethnic groups, it is important to remember that most people have two different alleles at each locus, and these vary among ethnic groups. Such differences make proper selection of donor material more important when tissue originates from a donor of different ethnic origin. The antigen A30, for example, runs in 30% of blacks, in only 1% of whites, and is absent in Japanese. On the other hand, the antigen, A9, occurs in 1% of blacks, 7% of whites, and 31% of Japanese.[31] According to Joysey, the dominant phenotype in England is HLA-A1, A2/H1 A8,1,12 (1%–2%). In Malaya, these antigens are rare, but antigens HLA-G and W15 are found in over 50% of the population. Tissue in this part of the world, therefore, is easier to match. Sharing of some antigens by different corneal donors (HLA-A2, 45% of European population) could explain infrequent second-graft reaction in patients with keratoconus (not second-set phenomena) and occasional bilateral rejections (second set).

The information just presented leads us to consider the *potential* acceptance of tissue grafts if they are perfectly compatible. Since such compatibility is far from being a reality, we must be satisfied with grafting tissues sharing some antigenic elements with the host, particularly when evidence in favor of tissue typing is not conclusive. It should be kept in mind, however, that in favor of tissue typing is the fact that autografts succeed in vascularized corneas, whereas allografts would fail.[39–47]

NONCOMPATIBILITY AND THE IMMUNE RESPONSE

When a full-thickness corneal transplant is sutured to the host cornea, the patient becomes the receptor of structures of molecular size (antigens) continuously elaborated and released by donor cells. These molecules can diffuse across the cornea and reach the lymphatic system in a matter of minutes or hours (see chapter 6). The same is true for antigens released by the graft endothelium into the aqueous humor. In this situation, we may have to consider the cornea as a portion of a large vessel (the uvea), in which a full-thickness graft, specifically its endothelium, would *not* be a privileged site as is suggested in the literature.

As we have previously seen, a high degree of allograft incompatibility does not mean that the graft will be rejected; however, the more dissimilar the tissue antigens are to those of the host, the more likely they are to incite the formation of antibodies. It is assumed that once the antigens reach the lymphatic circulation or the lymph node, they are captured by macrophages. In the lymph node, this cell will cause the *activation* of a certain population of lymphocytes. At this point, the lymphocytes have acquired the power to transfer sensitivity. According to Medawar,[46] peripheral lymphocytes can also be activated in contact with the antigen. These are the small, or the "T" (from thymus), lymphocytes that may originate clones of immunocompetent cells. They form the majority of circulating lymphocytes, the mediators of all hypersensitivities of the delayed type and the effectors of graft destruction.

The other type of lymphocytes, called "B" cells (from bursa), differ in origin, surface macromolecules, circulation pattern, and function[47] (see Table 5-2). The B lymphocytes have abundant immunoglobulin (IgG) molecules. However,

Table 5-2

Comparison of Mouse B and T Lymphocytes

Properties	B Cells	T Cells
Differentiation (from uncommitted Ag-insensitive "stem" cells to Ag-sensitive cells) in:	Bursa of Fabricius (in birds) or as yet unknown equivalent in mammals	Thymus
Ag-binding receptors on the cell surface:	Abundant Igs, (restricted to 1 isotype, 1 allotype, 1 idiotype per cell)	Nature of specific receptors is uncertain; Igs are sparse
Cell surface antigens:*		
θ	−	+
TL	−	+
Ly	−	+
PC	+ (plasma cells)	−
H-2 transplantation Ags	+	+
Approximate frequency (%) in:		
Blood	15	85
Lymph (thoracic duct)	10	90
Lymph node	15	85
Spleen	35	65
Bone marrow	Abundant	Few
Thymus	Rare	Abundant
Functions		
Secretion of antibody molecules	Yes (large lymphocytes and plasma cells)	No
Helper function (react with "carrier" moieties of the immunogen)	No	Yes
Effector cell for cell-mediated immunity	No	Yes
Distribution in lymph nodes and spleen:	Clustered in follicles around germinal centers	In interfollicular areas
Susceptibility to inactivation by:		
X-irradiation	++++	+
Corticosteroids	++	+
Antilymphocytic serum (ALS)	+	++++

Reproduced by permission.[47]

the T cells can become specifically sensitized to one antigen, and they can influence the differentiation of B cells into antibody-secreting plasma cells. Antibodies are proteins formed by lymphocytes and plasma cells in response to an antigen. They are serum proteins called immunoglobulins, also called 7-S Y-globulins, with a molecular weight of 150,000. Even though these immunoglobulins produced by some cells may not be directly responsible for graft destructions, there is evidence that, under certain circumstances, they may participate in allergic responses and complement fixation, and they may cause graft destruction in certain host corneal diseases.

REFERENCES

1. Erhlich P: Experimentelle Karzinomstudiem au Mausen. Arb Invest Exp Ther 1:77, 1906
2. Batchelor JR: Histocompatibility systems. Br Med J 21:100, 1965
3. Loeb L: Ueber Entstehirng eines Sarkom nach Transplantation eines Adenocarcinoms einer Japanischen Maus Z Krebsforsch 6:80, 1909
4. Little CC: A possible mendelian explanation for a type of inheritance apparently non-mendelian in nature. Science 40:904, 1914
5. Snell GD: Methods for the study of histocompatibility genes. J Genet 49:87, 1948
6. Woodruff MFA, Allan TM: Blood groups and the homograft problem. Br J Plast Surg 5:238, 1953
7. Klen R: Changes in Antibody Titers of the ABO and Rh Systems. II. Evaluation of 50 Cases. Csl Ophthal 11:246–249, 1955 Excerpta Medica (XII). 10:451, 1956
8. Nelken E, Nelken D, Michaelson IC, et al: ABO antigens in the human cornea. Nature 177:840, 1956
9. Ehlers N, Ahrons S: Corneal transplantation and histocompatibility. Acta Ophthalmol 49:513, 1971
10. Meyer HJ: Klinische und experimentele Untersuchungen zur Bedeutung von Iso-Antikorpern bei Keratoplastik. Habilitationsschrift, Gottingen. Bibl Ophthalmol 78:61, 1966
11. Mehri P, Becker B, Oglesby R: Corneal transplants and blood types: A clinical study. Am J Ophthalmol 47:48, 1959
12. Maumenee AE: The influence of donor–recipient sensitization on corneal grafts. Am J Ophthalmol 34:142, 1951
13. Maumenee AE: Clinical aspects of the corneal homograft reaction. Invest Ophthalmol 1:244, 1962
14. Bretscher MS: Direct lipid flow in all membranes. Nature 260:21, 1973
15. Schwartz BD, Natheuson SG: Regeneration of transplantation antigens on mouse cells. Transplant Proc 3:180, 1971
16. Joysey VC: Discussion: The influence of HL-A compatibility on the fate of corneal grafts, In Porter R,Knights J (eds): Corneal Graft Failure. Ciba Foundation Symposium. Elservier, Excerpta Medica, North-Holland, 1973, p 106
17. Medawar P: Immunity to homologous grafted skin III: The fate of skin homografts transplanted to the brain, to subcutaneous tissue, and the anterior chamber of the eye. Br J Exp Pathol 29:58, 1948
18. Woodruff MFA: The Transplantation of Tissues and Organs. Springfield, Ill, Charles C Thomas, 1960, p 401
19. Dempster WJ: The relationship between the antigen of skin and kidney of the dog. Br J Plast Surg 5:228, 1953

20. Ashwood-Smith MJ: Discussion: Difficulties in the use of tissue typing for corneal grafting, *In* Porter R, Knights J (eds): Corneal Graft Failure. Ciba Foundation Symposium. Elsevier, Excerpta Medica, North-Holland, 1973, p 337

21. Maumenee AE: The role of corneal vascularization in human corneal graft reactions, *In* Porter R, Knight J (eds): Corneal Graft Failure. Ciba Foundation Symposium. Elsevier, Excerpta Medica, North-Holland, 1973, pp 241–255

22. Fine M, Stein M: The role of corneal vascularization in human corneal graft reactions, *In* Porter R, Knight J (eds): Corneal Graft Failure. Ciba Foundation Symposium. Elsevier, Excerpta Medica, North-Holland, 1973, pp 193–208

23. Gibbs DC, Batchelor JR, Casey TA: The influence of HL-A compatibility on the fate of corneal grafts, *In* Porter R, Knight J (eds): Corneal Graft Failure. Ciba Foundation Symposium. Elsevier, Excerpta Medica, North-Holland, 1973, pp 293–306

24. Simonsen M, Buemann J, Gameltoft A, et al: Biological incompatibility in kidney transplantation in dogs. I. Experimental and morphological investigation. Acta Pathol Microbiol Scand 32:1, 1953

25. Hardin CA: Common antigenicity between skin grafts and total lung transplants. Transplant Bull 3:45, 1956

26. Khodadoust AA, Silverstein AM: Local graft-versus-host reaction within the anterior chamber of the eye: The formation of corneal endothelial pocks. Invest Ophthalmol 14:573, 1975

27. Khodadoust AA, Silverstein AM: Induction of corneal graft rejection by passive cell transfer. Invest Ophthalmol 15:89, 1976

28. Schaller JG, Omenn GS: The histocompatibility system and human disease. J Pediatr 88:913, 1976

29. Bach FH, van Rood JJ: The major histocompatibility complex. N Engl J Med 295:806, 1976

30. Meeting report of Sixth International Histocompatibility Testing Workshop, *In* Kissmeyer-Nielsen F (ed): Histocompatibility Testing, 1975. Copenhagen, Munksgaard, 1976

31. Bodmer WL: The HL-A System. Presented at the Johns Hopkins Centennial Symposium on Genetics, Baltimore, 1975

32. Stark WJ, Opelz G, Newsome D, et al: Sensitization to human lymphocyte antigens by corneal transplantation. Invest Ophthalmol 12:639, 1973

33. Allansmith MR, Fine M, Pryne R: Histocompatibility typing and corneal transplantation. Trans Am Acad Ophthalmol 78:445, 1974

34. Vannas S: Histocompatibility in corneal grafting. Invest Ophthalmol 14:883, 1975

35. Feldman JD: Immunological enhancement; A study of blocking antibodies. Adv Immunol 15:1679, 1972

36. Burde RM, Waltman SR, Berrios JM: Homograft rejection delayed by treatment of donor tissue in vitro with antilymphocytic serum. Science 173:921, 1971

37. Chandler JW, Gebhardt BM, Kaufman HE: Immunologic protection of rabbit corneal allografts: Preparation and in vitro testing of heterologous blocking antibody. Invest Ophthalmol 12:646, 1973

38. Binder PS, Gebhardt BM, Chandler JW, et al: Immunological protection of rabbit corneal allografts with heterologous blocking antibodies. Ann J Ophthalmol 14:469, 1975

39. Maumenee AE: Penetrating autokeratoplasty of entire cornea. Am J Ophthalmol 47:125, 1959

40. Barraquer J: Corneal autografting, *In* King JH, McTigue J (eds): The Cornea World Congress. Washington, Butterworths, 1965, pp 627–638

41. Elliot JH: Immunologic factor in penetrating keratoplasty, *In* Symposium on the Cornea. Transactions of the New Orleans Academy of Ophthalmology. St Louis, C. V. Mosby, 1972, p 68

42. Boruchoff A: Corneal autografts. Am J Ophthalmol 63:1677, 1967
43. Bundersen T, Calnan AF: Corneal autografts, ipsilateral and contralateral. Arch Ophthalmol 73:164, 1965
44. Vasco-Posada J: Ipsilateral autokeratoplasty. Am J Ophthalmol 64:717, 1967
45. Rycroft PV: Three unusual corneal grafts. Ophthalmol 41:759, 1957
46. Medawar PV: Transplantation of tissues and organs—Introduction. Br Med Bull 21:97, 1965
47. Eisen HN: Immunology, *In* Davis Dulbecco, Eisen et al (eds): Maryland, Harper and Row, 1973, pp 349–597

Chapter 6

The Antigenicity of Corneal Grafts

For many years it was accepted that the high rate of success of corneal grafts, when compared to other tissue grafts, was due not so much to the fact that the cornea was antigenically weak but because it was placed in a privileged avascular site.[1] It was believed also that graft survival was related to the barrier formed by the scar tissue[2] or to the high mucopolysaccharide content of the cornea.[3] Since it was learned that grafts could succumb to an immune reaction, cellular and noncellular antigens have been searched for. In the past, these studies were not very rewarding with allografts, in part because the immunologic techniques were not sensitive enough to detect antibodies generated by allografts. Until recently, it had been suspected that antigen release from a graft occurred only after cell death; but we have seen in Chapter 5 that cells can release antigens from the surface and elaborate them again. The presence of noncellular antigens was suspected, since incubation of xenografts for several hours decreased its antigenicity.[4,5] These antigens present in the ground substance were identified by Robert et al.[6] and shown by Remky,[7] but they were antigenic only within a xenograft system. Whereas it is possible that the antigens in the ground substance of xenografts could diminish by incubation or soaking, in allografts, this (unproven) reduction in antigenicity could be related to cell death. In human transplants, Stocker[8] found a rise or development of antibodies during graft rejection by the method of mixed hemaglutination. Nelken and Nelken[25] also found anticorneal antibodies in 13 of 33 grafted patients using a similar method. These results have not been confirmed by others. Immunologic studies on corneal heterografts by several authors[9–17] indicated that the epithelium was the most antigenic layer of the cornea and that after its removal, xenografts could survive. These observations influenced the custom of removing the epithelium from donor corneas at the time of transplantation in order to diminish their antigenicity.[8] In 1952, Choyce[18] reported successful transplantation of lamellar xenografts (human and cat to rabbit) after epithelial removal. His experiments were repeated by others with similar results, proving that in some circumstances, corneal xenografts could be accepted and remain clear, but they did not demonstrate that this tissue, with its epithelium removed, lacked antigenicity. Destruction by freezing of corneal cells did not seem to reduce the antigenicity of intralamellar corneal pig transplants in rabbits, as was demonstrated by Lorenzetti and Kaufman in 1966.[19] In their experiment, frozen and thawed pig corneas induced histologic rejection, and these transplants were destroyed simultaneously with fresh pig xenografts. In 1973, Townsend, Polack, and Slappey[20] showed that cryopreserved xenografts also behaved like fresh xenografts when placed intralamellarly in rabbit corneas. The relative antigenic importance of the three corneal layers was studied. It was observed that the intralamellar transplantation of cryopreserved pig corneas demonstrated a higher reaction when corneal epithelium was included. On the other hand, Shultz and Gallun[21] found that when cryopreserved dog corneas were placed intralamellarly in the rabbit eye, they did not produce an immune reaction, as was found when fresh tissue was implanted. They concluded that the cryopreservation technique did modify the antigenicity of the donor cornea as a result of freezing or by the use of the cryoprotective solutions. We found, however, that fresh rabbit corneas were well tolerated by cat corneas when placed intralamellarly,[22] and even small fish-to-rabbit xenografts (personal observation)[23] were viable. I believe that in addition to the antigenic response, which is greater the farther away from the zoologic scale, the large size (antigenic dose) and thickness (mechanical disruption) of a xenograft favors vascularization and rejection. Our clinical experience shows that cryopreserved human corneas are subject to tissue reactions similar to fresh tissue when partial- or full-thickness grafts are performed. Experiments with heterografts, therefore, must be cautiously evaluated. Billingham and Boswell, in 1953,[1] and Khodadoust and Silverstein, in 1966,[23] showed that corneal epithelium growing on a vascularized skin site on the rabbit, but not invaded by vessels, were subjected to the rejection mechanism. In carefully controlled studies, Khodadoust and Silverstein (1969)[24] showed that each type of corneal cell is capable of inducing host sensitization and rejection. It is well known at the present time that in the human, corneal transplants may show destruction of endothelial, stromal, or epithelial cells at once or separately.

Interstitial or ground substance may also sensitize the host, but only if this is a xenograft.[25] This interstitial substance is produced by the liberation of serum proteins in the tissue, especially the neutral glycoproteins (glycosaminoglycans).[26] According to Offret and Pouliquen,[26] the incubation of corneal tissue in serum with the purpose of decreasing its antigenicity may have some effect with xenografts but not allografts, since these proteins are not antigenic within the same species. The question was also raised of whether blood antigens influenced graft survival. Several reports in favor and against the influence of ABO antigens on graft rejection have been published; for example, Klen, in 1955,[22] and Nelken et al., 1957,[28] reported a rise in isoaglutinins after ABO-incompatible transplantation. Alberth, in 1958,[29] also observed some correlation in cases of incompatible blood group transplantation. In our experience, that of Ehlers and Ahrons in 1971,[30] and that of Meyer in 1968,[31] there was no significant correlation between corneal transplantation results and blood group incompatibility. According to Ehlers and Ahrons,[30] this lack of consistency is not surprising, because ABO compatibility is only one of the many factors that may influence graft rejection in addition to the HLA antigens. Other factors are the status of the host, the size of the graft, etc.

As previously mentioned, corneal grafts contain minor (noncellular) and major (cellular) histocompatibility antigens. Noncellular antigens are contained in the stromal tissue, from where they may easily diffuse out of the graft to mix with the host intrastromal fluid. The antigens may then leave the host cornea by perilimbal lymphatics; however, some authors believe that macrophages or lymphoid cells may carry antigens from the corneal to the lymphatic channels.

We have been able to confirm the observation of Collin[32] and Pouliquen[33] that vascularized host corneas contain new lymphatic channels.

There is another subject of interest that concerns the time required by a graft to initiate the sensitization process, or how soon antigens can leave the graft and be captured by the host reticuloendothelial tissue. The practical importance of these phenomena supports the use of steroids or immunosuppressive drugs very early after grafting. There is evidence that in kidney grafting, immunosuppressive drugs must be used before or at the time of surgery if immunosuppression is to be obtained.[34] In our experiments with heterografts, we found that host sensitization to intralamellar xenografts develops as soon as 1 hr after intralamellar keratoplasty.

Polack and Bowman[35] studied the period of time for an intralamellar pig xenograft to be rejected when placed in a rabbit eye. Two types of experiments were performed (Fig. 6-1). In the first study, a graft that included epithelium was

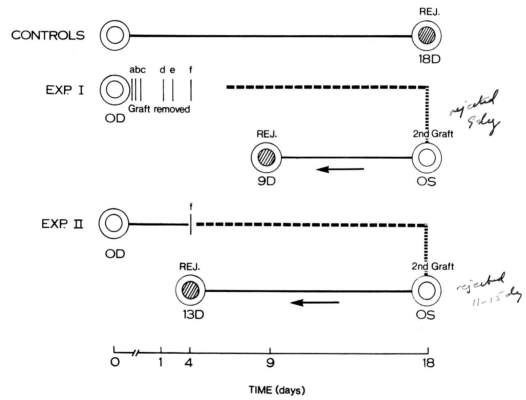

Figure 6-1. Intralamellar xenografts reject 18 days after keratoplasty. In experiment I, intralamellar xenografts were removed after implantation at 1, 2, or 4 hr after surgery (**A, B,** and **C**) or they were removed at 1, 2, and 4 days (**D, E,** and **F**). Eighteen days following this surgery, a second intralamellar graft was placed in the unoperated eye, and this rejected at 9 days. The tissue used for the second graft was a portion of the same donor tissue used for the first graft, which had been preserved by freezing. In experiment II, a similar procedure was done; however, the second graft was tissue from an unrelated donor. This graft was rejected between 11 and 15 days.

placed in the right eye of each experimental rabbit, and the wound was sutured. The graft remained in situ for periods of time that varied from 1, 2, and 4 hr or 1, 2, and 4 days after keratoplasty. At that time, the transplant was removed, and the cornea was resutured. Eighteen to 22 days later, a second implant was placed in the opposite eye, again using the same corneal tissue that had been preserved. In all rabbits in which the second graft (second set) from the same donor was implanted, the average rejection time was 9 days. The average rejection time for a first-set intralamellar xenograft rejection was 18 days. Rabbits that had been exposed to a graft for only 1 or 2 hr had rejected the second graft at 11 days; however, those exposed to the first graft for longer periods of time rejected the transplant within 1 wk. In a control experiment, the second transplant was obtained from unrelated donor material and was rejected between 11 and 15 days. These experiments showed that host sensitization to an intralamellar corneal graft starts as soon as the graft is placed in the recipient cornea, even though avascular. Antigens must have reached the corneal limbus by diffusion through the corneal lamellae on their way to the local lymphoid area or regional lymphatic nodes. Sensitization to this type of graft does not require that the host cornea be vascularized or that host lymphocytes should reach the graft to pick up antigens. It is possible, however, that vascularized host corneas could become sensitized in a shorter period of time or that sensitization of higher degree could develop. An argument against this study would be that epithelial or endothelial cells from the graft might have been left in situ after removing the graft, thus acting as a continuous source of antigens; but the amount of cells that detached from these intralamellar grafts might have been very small to act as a potent antigenic source. These experimental studies do not prove that a similar type of sensitization may develop in human homologous transplantation, but it supports the theory of an intrastromal pathway for antigen diffusion in avascular corneas.

REFERENCES

1. Billingham RE, Boswell T: Studies on the problem of corneal homografts. Proc Roy Soc Lond (Biol) 141:392, 1953
2. Duke ES: The problem of homoplastic grafting as applied to the cornea. J R Coll Surg Edinb 1:187, 1955
3. Bacshich P, Wyburn GM: The significance of the muco protein content on the survival of homografts of cartilage and cornea. Proc Roy Soc Edinb (Biol) 62:321, 1947
4. Geeraets WJ, Chan G, Guerry D: Corneal Antigenicity. Immuno electrophonetic study. Arch Ophthalmol 64:413, 1960
5. Stocker FW, Matton van Leuwen MT, Georgiade N: Host tissue reaction to fresh and frozen corneas. Am J Ophthalmol 53:279, 1962
6. Robert L, Payrau P, Pouliquen Y, et al: Role of a structural glycoprotein of corneal stroma in transplantation immunity. Nature 207:383, 1965
7. Remky H: Le conflit immunologique dans l'heterogreffe de cornee etudes experimentalles. Comparison des cornees fraiches et silico-deseches. Bull Mem Soc Fr Ophthalmol 75:210, 1962
8. Stocker RW: Soluble antigens and isoantibodies, *In* Rycroft PV (ed): Corneo-plastic Surgery. London, Pergamon, 1967, p 152
9. Paul SD: Hetero-corneal transplantation in experimental rabbits. Ophthalmologica 147:334, 1964

10. Sykes JH, Girard LG: Heterologous corneal transplants in rabbits. Am J Ophthalmol 48:259, 1959

11. Basu PK, Ormsby, HL: Corneal heterografts in rabbits. Am J Ophthalmol 44:477, 1957

12. Tsutsui J, Watanabe S, Murakami N: Lyophilized cornea in experimental heterografts. Am J Ophthalmol 54:265, 1962

13. Lieb WA, Lerman S: Keratoplasty and allergic reactions. Klin Monatsbl Augenheilkd 132:31, 1958

14. Babel J, Bourqin JB: Experimental research with corneal heterografts. Br J Ophthalmol 36:529, 1952

15. Tsuitsui J, Watanabe S: Corneal heterografts of fish cornea into rabbit eyes. Am J Ophthalmol 48:363, 1959

16. Kuwahara, Y: Studies on heterotransplantation of corneas. Am J Ophthalmol 53:911, 1962

17. Agarwal LP, Mohan M: Intralamellar corneal heterograft of frog cornea into rabbit cornea. Br J Ophthalmol 47:14, 1963

18. Choyce DP: Successful transplantation of human and cat corneal tissue into rabbit cornea. Br J Ophthalmol 36:537, 1952

19. Lorenzetti DWC, Kaufman HE: Experimental production of graft reactions with suppression by topical steroids. Arch Ophthalmol 76:274, 1966

20. Townsend W, Polack FM, Slappey T: Antigenicity of fresh and cryopreserved xenografts, In Capella JA (ed): Corneal Preservation. Springfield Ill, Charles C Thomas, 1973, pp 294–299

21. Schultz RO, Gallun AB: The effects of cryopreservation on the corneal heterograft reaction, In Capella JA (ed): Corneal Preservation. Springfield Ill, Charles C Thomas, 1973, pp 300–307

22. Polack FM, Smelser GK, Rose J: The fate of cells in heterologous corneal transplants. Invest Ophthalmol 2:355, 1963

23. Khodadoust AA, Silverstein AM: Studies on the heterotopic transplantation of cornea to the skin, In Hanna C (ed): Symposium on Suppression of Graft Rejection with Emphasis on the Cornea. Baltimore, Williams & Wilkins, 1966, pp 435–443

24. Khodadoust AA, Silverstein AM: The survival and rejection of epithelium in experimental corneal grafts. Invest Ophthalmol 8:169, 1969

25. Robert L, Payrau P, Pouliquen Y, et al: Role of a structural glycoprotein of corneal stroma in transplantation immunity. Nature 207:383, 1965

26. Offret G, Pouliquen Y, Guyot D: Aspects cliniques des reactions immunitaires apres keratoplasties transfixiantes chez L'homme. Arch Ophthalmol (Paris) 30:209, 1970

27. Klen R: Changes in antibody titres of the ABO and RH systems. II. Evaluation of 50 cases. Csl Ophthalmol 11:246, cited in Excerpta Medica, Section XII, 10:451, 1955

28. Nelken E, Nelken D, Michaelson IC, et al: ABO antigens in the human cornea. Nature 177:840, 1956

29. Alberth B: Surgical treatment of caustic injuries of the eye. Budapest, Akademiai Kaido, 1968

30. Ehlers N, Ahrons S: Corneal transplantation and histocompatibility. Acta Ophthalmol 49:513, 1971

31. Meyer HJ: Zum Nachweis von serum-antikorpern nach Keratoplastik. Albrecht von Graefes Arch Klin Ophthalmol 176:283, 1968

32. Collin HB: Lymphatic drainage of I131 albumin from the vascularized cornea. Invest Ophthalmol 9:146, 1970

33. Faure JP, Kozak Y, Graf B, et al: Lymphatiques dans la corneé vascularisee au cours du reject d'heterogreffes experimentales. Arch Ophthalmol (Paris) 30:575, 1970

34. Starzl TE: Problems in renal homotransplantation. JAMA 738:734, 1964

35. Polack FM, Bowman B: Time period for intralamellar heterograft sensitization. Presented at A.R.V.O. meeting, Sarasota, April 1973

Chapter 7

Basic Problems in Corneal Grafting

In spite of the many advances in corneal graft instrumentation, surgical techniques, and handling of the donor tissue, we can still identify mechanical and biologic problems as two main causes of graft failure. It is well known that most of the mechanical problems (poor coaptation, suture malposition, ectasia, leakage, synechiae, etc.) leading to graft failure occur at the time of surgery or in the early postoperative days. Once the graft has been fixed to the host by scar tissue, problems related to wound apposition or sutures will sharply decrease, while biologic problems tend to increase.

Minimize tissue handling in order to preserve as much endothelium as possible is rule number one if we are to reduce the magnitude of postoperative graft edema and mechanical problems. Even though the importance of the corneal endothelium was recognized several years ago, only recently have we become aware of the functional reserve of this corneal layer through its study with the specular microscope. It was known that the number of endothelial cells was greater in the young than in older persons.[1,2] Minimal importance was given to this fact because most grafts were obtained from eyes of older persons, and there were no differences in results of keratoplasties from these donors provided they appeared normal under the slit lamp. Young, normal corneas have about 5000 endothelial cells per square millimeter;[3] but while some old corneas have small drop in cell population, others show a significant reduction even though they are clinically normal. Specular microscopic studies by Forstot and Kaufman[4] have shown that after an apparently uncomplicated and atraumatic intraocular procedure, there is a consistent and significant loss of endothelial cells. In keratoplasty, this loss may rise to 50% and may be the cause of irreversible edema of the graft (usually called "primary tissue failure") if the donor tissue had a very low cell population. Other unrecognized problems can be handled adequately today by screening donor eyes with the specular microscope. Two additional rules are: use fine and adequate instruments under microscopic magnification and suture material as deep as possible to approximate better the posterior wound. In regards to suture material, the use of fine silk (9′ 0′) or nylon sutures (9′ 0′ and 10′ 0′) is almost mandatory today, because the amount of inflammatory reaction induced is minimal when compared to older sutures, such as the 6′ 0′ and 7′ 0′ silk. In selected cases, the use of 8′ 0′ silk may be indicated; however, in vascularized corneas, where we prefer not to increase the inflammatory response, we can solve the problem using the more inert synthetic sutures and steroids.

Some trauma to the donor tissue cannot be avoided, but must be minimized.

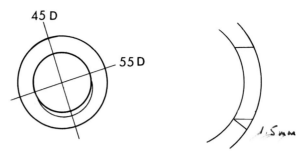

Figure 7-1. Schema indicating Troutman's wedge resection procedure to reduce post-operative corneal astigmatism. The resection of 1.5 mm of corneal stroma in 2 hr of the clock at 90° to the steeper meridian reduces 5–8 diopters.

In my opinion, the posterior or endothelial cut of the graft is superior to the anterior cut because it is less traumatic and its edges are more regular.

High astigmatism in a clear graft is a frustrating (although infrequent) complication, since spectacles or contact lenses are unsatisfactory to correct this refractive error. These astigmatic defects however can be corrected or reduced with the "wedge resection" of Troutman[5] (Fig. 7-1).

The real basic problems that we are being confronted with at the present time are those related to the homograft reaction, control of graft vascularization, modification of biologic situations that may affect the transparency of the graft (such as increased intraocular pressure or inflammation), and the possible effect of vitreous contact on recent grafts in aphakic eyes. An equally serious problem is that related to the growth of retrocorneal fibrous membranes, usually present in eyes with severe chemical burns or in eyes with repeated corneal surgery. We are just beginning to explore the different ways to alter or modify the biologic problems of the graft reaction through adequate tissue typing or by the use of immunosuppressive agents, but we are far from being able to control all the other problems mentioned.

Ultramicroscopic studies of pathologic corneas have provided useful information about the nature of the disease, its localization, and potential for recurrence. However, morphological evidence has not been of much help in some conditions, such as chemical burns, dry eyes, and severe herpetic disease, which are still problem cases for transplantation. As we shall see in future chapters, in some instances, we may be able to improve the basic disease in order to improve the graft prognosis.

REFERENCES

1. Irvine AR, Irvine AR Jr: Variations in normal human corneal endothelium. Am J Ophthalmol 36:1272–1285, 1953
2. Kaufman HE, Capella JA, Robbins JE: The corneal endothelium. Am J Ophthalmol 61:835, 1966

3. Bourne WM, Kaufman HE: Specular microscopy of human corneal endothelium in vivo. Am J Ophthalmol 81:319, 1976
4. Forstot SL, Blackwell WL, Jaffe NS, et al: The effect of intraocular lens implantation on the corneal endothelium. Trans Am Acad Ophthalmol Otolaryngol 83:195, 1977
5. Troutman RC: Cataract survey of the cataract—Phacoemulsification committee. Trans Am Acad Ophthalmol Otolaryngol 70:178, 1975

Chapter 8

Donor Tissue

Donor eyes, donor tissue, or donor corneas are terms used interchangeably. In recent years, important changes have occurred in the methods of corneal preservation for penetrating keratoplasties that have revolutionized corneal transplantation.[1-6]

The removal of eyes and transportation to the eye bank is the first step in the sequence of events that terminates in a corneal graft. For years, time has been the most critical element in obtaining satisfactory tissue for penetrating kerato-plasty, since the donor cornea deteriorated while the eye was kept in a moist chamber at +4°C. Whereas today we demand corneas obtained less than 10 hr post-mortem, in the past, some authors have preferred the use of corneas after 48 hr.[7-11] The newer techniques of tissue preservation have extended the time corneas can be kept in storage, which at present varies from several days (short-term) to months (cryopreservation).

In most countries, eyes are distributed to surgeons through eye banks. It is their responsibility to deliver eyes with adequate medical information so the surgeon can decide if the donor tissue qualifies for his patient. The eye banks also have the responsibility of delivering safe eyes from the bacteriologic point of view. This important aspect of eye banking starts at the time of enucleation, which must be done under aseptic conditions, and continues through the storage procedure until the cornea is used.

ENUCLEATION OF THE EYE

Instruments Required

Speculum, 1 fixation forceps, 1 fine forceps (Bishop-Harmon), 2 mosquito forceps, strabismus scissors, enucleation scissors, strabismus hook, needle holder, 4' 0' silk, cotton balls, and a syringe of irrigating saline solution.

Technique

After placing the speculum in the eye, the cornea and conjunctiva are irrigated with normal saline solution, and several drops of an antibiotic solution (Neosporin ®) are applied to the cornea. With a fine forceps and the strabismus scissors, the conjunctiva is separated from the limbus in 360°, and the tissue is undermined. The scissors are introduced through Tenon's capsule, applying them close to the sclera. A cleavage plane is obtained, which is spread out between the recti muscles posteriorly towards the optic nerve. This procedure is performed around the circumference of the globe until all conjunctiva and Tenon's capsule is separated, and the muscles are visible. With a muscle hook, the muscles are identified, lifted, and cut with the strabismus scissors, leaving 3 – 4 mm of muscle tendon attached to the sclera. The four recti muscles are sectioned, as well as the oblique muscles. While the eye is being lifted by the medial and lateral recti with mosquito clamps, all remaining adhesions between the globe and Tenon's capsule are cut by spreading the enucleation scissors, which are then introduced to the posterior pole of the globe from the temporal side to cut the optic nerve. The eye is lifted, all remaining attachments to Tenon's are cut, and the globe is deposited on a sterile towel. Here it is again rinsed with saline and placed on a sterile eye holder and in a moist chamber. Enough cotton is introduced into the orbital socket to produce an adequate cosmetic appearance of the eyelids. Usually no conjunctival sutures are required.

EXCISION OF THE CORNEA

In some instances, enucleation of the globe is not permitted, while permission can be obtained to remove the cornea with a scleral rim. In this case, similar aseptic techniques are employed; the eye lids are spread with a speculum and the conjunctival fornices are rinsed with saline solution. With a fine forceps and strabismus scissors, the conjunctiva is separated from its limbal insertion, the globe is grasped with a fixation forceps, and with a Bard-Parker #15 blade, the sclera is incised 3 mm from the limbus until the choroidal tissue is visible. The opening must be 5 – 10 mm in length so a scissors can be inserted between the sclera and the suprachoroidal space. The cornea is gently lifted and separated from the iris (this is a very important step, since Descemet's membrane can be detached from the cornea if the maneuver is done abruptly), and then it is immersed in a short-term preservation solution (M-K media).

A large trephine (11 mm) can also be used for the corneal excision. The eye is immobilized preferentially with two fixation forceps. Then the surgeon or an assistant applies the trephine, properly centered, and cuts the cornea without excessive pressure on the globe (the procedure works better if the trephine is electrically or mechanically powered). If the cornea is not completely cut with the trephine, the section is completed with forceps and fine scissors. These corneas are immediately immersed into the M-K preservation media.

Figure 8-1A–F shows the various steps of corneal excision from an enucleated eye as done routinely in our Eye Bank or in the operating room.

BACTERIOLOGY OF EYE BANK EYES

The contamination of donor eyes with pathogen microorganisms has always been of great concern to eye surgeons. It has been established that the incidence of bacterial contamination of the normal human conjunctiva has slight variation around the world. Rollins and Stocker[12] also found that the conjunctival flora of donor eyes shows no bacterial growth. In a study we did in 1967,[13] in which 240 eye bank eyes were cultured, we found 100% positive cultures, and with few exceptions, we found that the bacterial flora of enucleated eyes was similar to

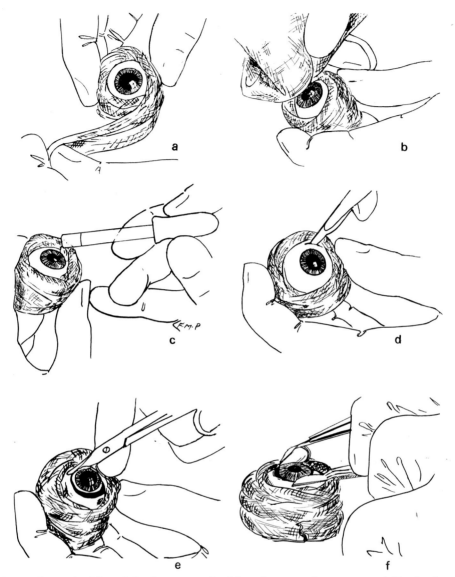

Figure 8-1. A. The globe is wrapped with a long sterile gauze and **B.** the loose epithelium is removed with a gauze. **C.** Antibiotic drops are applied several times to the corneal surface. **D.** The sclera is incised 3 mm from the limbus. **E.** With blunt scissors, the cornea is excised with a scleral rim. **F.** The cornea is gently lifted from the eye, while the iris is held back with a blade.

that of normal conjunctiva. These exceptions were mostly due to the high incidence of gram-negative organisms (Table 8-1).

A high incidence of positive cultures is probably related to the method of culturing and isolation. The cultures obtained from the surface of the cornea or sclera were taken in the bacteriology laboratory, so the plating or broth inoculation was made immediately. In all of these eyes, the surface of the globe was

Table 8-1
Sensitivity of Microorganisms Isolated From "Donor" Eyes*

Antibiotics Nitrofurans Sulfonamides	S. aureus Percent Sensitive	Klebsiella Group Percent Sensitive	E. coli Percent Sensitive	Proteus Group Percent Sensitive	P. aeruginosa Percent Sensitive
Ampicillin	—	30.8	50.0	37.5	—
Bacitracin	85.5	—	—	—	—
Chloramphenicol (Chloromycetin)	83.1	51.0	73.9	90.0	40.0
Cephalothin	91.2	76.9	75.0	75.0	—
Colistin sulfate	—	75.5	60.9	10.0	100
Dimethoxyphenyl-penicillin	83.1	—	—	—	—
Dihydrostrepto-mycin	68.7	49.0	60.9	50.0	10.0
Erythromycin	84.3	—	—	—	—
Nitrofurazone	90.4	77.6	87.0	90.0	30.0
Sulfisoxazole (Gantrisin)	9.6	6.1	8.7	10.0	—
Kanamycin sulfate (Kantrex)	88.0	51.0	56.5	80.0	—
Lincomycin	97.7	—	—	—	—
Neomycin	92.8	79.6	91.3	90.0	40.0
Novobiocin	90.4	51.0	60.0	20.0	10.0
Penicillin	63.9	—	—	—	—
Polymyxin B	—	87.8	65.2	10.0	100
Sodium oxacillin (Prostaphlin)	85.7	—	—	—	—
Sulfadiazine	9.6	6.1	8.7	10.0	10.0
Tetracycline	61.5	57.1	87.0	20.0	30.0

*The few streptococci and pneumococci found proved to be sensitive to chloramphenicol erythromycin, nitrofurazone, penicillin, and tetracycline.
Reproduced by permission.[13]

cleaned with sterile cotton applicators moistened with trypticase soy broth, and inoculations were made in blood-agar and chocolate-agar plates, thioglycollate broth and Sabouraud dextrose agar plates. The following methods for reducing or eliminating bacteria were tested:

1. Thimerosol, merthiolate (solution 1:5000)—four eyes were soaked in this solution, and cultures were done after 15, 40, or 45 min of immersion.
2. Benzalkonium chloride (1:1000—two eyes were immersed for 15 min in this solution, and four eyes were immersed for 30 min.
3. Benzalkonium chloride (1:1000) and ultrasound cleaning for 1 min—the stainless steel cups of an ultrasound cleaning machine were sterilized and filled with benzalkonium chloride (1:1000) in which six eyes were treated for 1 min. Cultures were done following a saline rinse after the treatment.

4. Ethylene-oxide gas—four eyes were placed in the container of an ethylene-oxide gas sterilizer for 4 hr before culturing.
5. Polymyxin B, neomycin, and gramicidin (Neosporin) solution drip for 2 min over the cornea—22 eyes were treated in this fashion before cultures were repeated.
6. Removal of corneal epithelium—14 eye bank eyes were wrapped in sterile gauze, except for the cornea, and the corneal epithelium was rubbed off in one direction only with another sterile gauze, trying to use a sterile portion of the gauze at the time. The partially denuded cornea was then cultured.

The result of corneal cultures after immersion of the globe for 15 min in the merthiolate solution produced more colonies than before immersion. This was interpreted as recontamination of the globe with its own bacteria from a medium that was bacteriostatically ineffective. Additional treatment for another 30 min in a change of the same antiseptic solution failed to sterilize the eye. Immersion in benzalkonium chloride for 15 min showed a decrease in bacterial growth, and sterilized the corneal tissue after 30 min; however, the epithelium had by then sloughed off completely, and the corneal stroma had become hazy. When ultrasound was combined with the immersion in benzalkonium chloride, sterilization of the globe was also obtained; but because of destruction of the epithelial surface, we examined the endothelium with nitro blue tetrazolium (NBT) stains. The endothelium of all of these eyes had become permeable to the NBT dye, indicating damage of this layer by the ultrasound or the antiseptic solution.

Sterilization with ethylene oxide produced similar changes in the endothelial layer, even though the surface of the cornea produced negative cultures. Frequent dripping of Neosporin solution on the cornea for a period of 2 min gave satisfactory results. We found that it was impossible to sterilize the whole globe by immersion in this solution; therefore, we decided to consider the sclera as contaminated tissue and keep it isolated from the cornea while it was bathed in the antibiotic solution. Of 22 eyes studied in this group, 6 gave positive cultures, but the number of colonies was minimal when compared with the pretreatment culture. The removal of corneal epithelium also gave a marked decrease in the number of colonies present in the cornea. Only 3 of 13 eyes treated this way gave negative cultures, but the other 10 showed a marked decrease in the number of colonies (Table 8-2).

The method we recommend, therefore, is the treatment of the globe with the antibiotic solution immediately after enucleation when the globes are sent to the eye bank. Just before processing for M-K media or before being used for surgery, the loose or dead corneal epithelium should be gently removed with sterile gauze (Fig. 8-1B), trying not to use the same material twice over the cornea. Following this, the cornea should be treated with frequent drops of the Neosporin solution for a period of about 2 min (Fig. 8-1C). This treatment assures a minimal survival of bacterial contaminants. However, no perfect sterility of corneal tissue will ever be guaranteed. We have found that treatment with the mixture of polymyxin B, neomycin and gramicidin is one of the most effective, and our findings were in agreement with those of Doctor and Hughes,[14] Paton,[15] and Rollins and Stocker,[12] who recommended irrigation of the donor eye with saline solution at the time of enucleation and subsequent treatment with the antibiotic solution.

Table 8-2
Bacterial Colonies in Donor Eyes

Agent	Time	Before	After	Tissue Damage	Number of Eyes
Thimerosol solution 1:5000	15 min	++	+++	0	4
	30 min	++	++	+	
	45 min	++	+	++	
Benzalkonium chloride	15 min	++	+	+	2
1:1000	30 min	++	+−	++	4
Benzalkonium and ultrasound	1 min	++	0	+++	6
Ethylene oxide	2 hr	++	0	+++	4
Neosporin	2 min	++	−+	0	22
Removal of corneal epithelium	−	++	−+	0	14
N.S. Irrigation plus epithelium removal plus Neosporin (2 hr)	−	++	0	0	12

Reproduced by permission.[13]
  CODE: No growth = 0; occasional colony = +−; Few colonies = +; numerous colonies = ++ or +++

SUITABILITY OF DONOR MATERIAL

The large demand of donor tissue for corneal transplantation has stimulated the development of improved ways to extend the storage time, and new ways of preservation have been devised so corneas can now be used several days or months after removal, depending on the type of storage technique. Research along these lines also has determined the optimal qualifications for donor tissue to be considered of prime quality. This has resulted in better clinical results which, however, cannot be separated from parallel improvements in instrumentation and technique.

Age

It has been shown in previous chapters that transplanted endothelial tissue persists almost indefinitely in adequate hosts (chapter 2); one clinical example is that of persistent clear grafts in corneal endothelial dystrophies. For this reason, the ideal donor tissue is a young cornea, since it has a larger number of endothelial cells. An inevitable loss of endothelial cells during surgery will not affect the survival of these grafts. Unfortunately, most of the corneas obtained for transplantation fall between the ages of 60 and 80, with an average age of 70

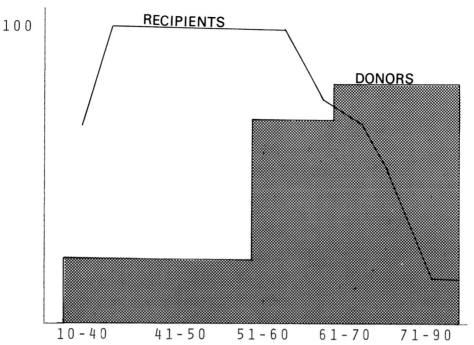

Figure 8-2. Graph showing the age distribution and availability of donor eyes at the North Florida Eye Bank.

yr. Recipients, however, are on the average 15 – 20 yr younger than the donors (Fig. 8-2). Donor corneas of advanced age require more careful screening to detect possible cornea guttata or unusual increased thickness, as well as the number of cells that can be determined with the specular microscope. Grafts with a low number of endothelial cells have a higher risk of failure. It has been estimated by Bourne and Kaufman[16] that there is a 30%–40% endothelial cell loss following keratoplasty, the loss being more pronounced in phakic than in aphakic cases.

We prefer to match the age of the donor with that of the recipient as close as possible if several donor corneas are available; however, corneas from old donors without pathology, or with an average number of cells, are excellent donor tissue. The presence of arcus senilis is not a contraindication for its use, but it will limit the size of the graft, mostly for aesthetic reasons. Very young corneas (less than 2 yr) are not usually obtained and seem to be rather thin for use in adult eyes. Corneas from donors of 2–5 years of age are suitable tissue, but they have a higher curvature, which in some instances can be used to correct high hyperopia.

Time Post Mortem

The period of time elapsed between death and enucleation and storage at 4°C or preservation are important factors for endothelial cell survival. Age is another factor, as well as cause of death in some instances. A recent survey by

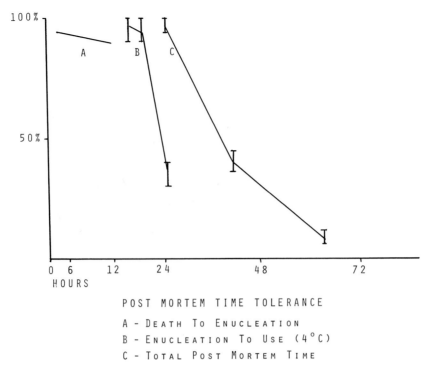

POST MORTEM TIME TOLERANCE

A – DEATH TO ENUCLEATION

B – ENUCLEATION TO USE (4°C)

C – TOTAL POST MORTEM TIME

Figure 8-3. Post mortem time tolerance for usability of donor eyes. **A.** Most surgeons will accept eyes removed within 12 hr. **B.** Some will use eyes stored up to 20 hr; about 40% will accept them up to 24 hr. **C.** Few surgeons will use eyes with total postmortem time (**A** + **B**) exceeding 26 hr. Fewer surgeons still will use eyes totalling 60 hr (**A** + **B**).

McCarey et al.[17] indicated that a large proportion of surgeons preferred corneal tissue that had been removed before 12 hr. It should be noted, however, that many eye banks are now obtaining tissue before 6 hr post mortem. After storage at 4°C, most surgeons will not use corneas beyond 24 hr, and few will not use them past 48 hr. The subject of corneal tissue viability is discussed later in this chapter. (Fig. 8-3)

Cause of Death and Donor Conditions Unsuitable for Grafting

Even though there is no specific information about the effect of antimitotic drugs on corneal tissue, we have the clinical impression that corneas from patients with cancer who have been treated with immunosuppressive drugs do not survive cryopreservation and do not function as well as tissue from healthy donors after transplantation. Chromosomal alterations have been found by Dr. J. Frias of the University of Florida in limited experiments of cultured rabbit corneal stromal cells after treatment with Cytoxan. The same impression is obtained when donor tissue has been obtained from debilitated donors.[18] In the same survey by McCarey et al. in 1975, the following answers were obtained on questionnaires sent to eye surgeons and eye banks:

1. Evaluation of Donor Eyes (by Eye Banks)
    A. Slit Lamp   77%
    B. Gross appearance   29%
    C. Corneal thickness   17%
    D. Other   17%
2. Cultures
    Yes   31%   No   63%
3. Corneas Not Acceptable for Grafting (by Surgeons)
    A. Hepatitis   97%
    B. Anterior segment tumors   83%
    C. Septicemia   74%
    D. Retinoblastoma   60%
    E. Aphakia   69%
    F. Syphilis   57%
    G. Glaucoma   57%
    H. Leukemia   54%
    I. Ca , on antimetabolites
    J. Debilitation.

VIABILITY OF CORNEAL TISSUE

It is well known today that viability of corneal tissue for penetrating keratoplasty depends almost exclusively on the survival of corneal endothelial cells. Years ago, it was considered that viability of corneal tissue depended on the survival of corneal stromal cells, and it was estimated by the metabolic rate of this tissue.[19] To a great extent, when we examine eye bank eyes with the slit lamp prior to corneal storage or preservation, we are measuring the degree of endothelial permeability (alterations) and corneal edema. Shortly after death, before corneal edema develops and stromal folds appear, it is impossible to determine if the endothelial layer has abnormal cells or guttata formation. According to King,[19] significant loss of corneal transparency occurs as soon as 4 hr after death, and stromal edema, with folds in Descemet's membrane, appears at 48–72 hr after death. Stocker et al.[20] described profound endothelial damage after 4 days of storage at +4°C. From the ultrastructural point of view, endothelial as well as stromal and epithelial cell changes start shortly after death. They were described by Shaeffer in 1963[21] and more recently by Van Horn and Shultz.[22] These observations, as well as histologic studies and biomicroscopic examination of enucleated eyes, can only be taken as a baseline for alterations that may develop in most eye bank eyes. The problem is that there are too many variables in human eyes to describe similar changes in a series of eyes of similar age. Morphological alterations of endothelial cells vary markedly between eye donors because their fatal disease or a prolonged agony may affect the endothelial cells,[18] as may the medication used before death. The room temperature where the cadaver was kept before the eyes were removed also has an influence on the cell survival, as does the time elapsed between death and enucleation.

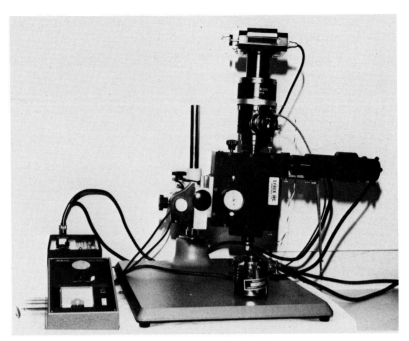

Figure 8-4. The specular microscope manufactured by Syber Co., Gainesville, Fla.

SPECULAR MICROSCOPY

The most promising method to evaluate donor corneas is by examining the corneal endothelium with the specular microscope (Fig. 8-4). This microscope, first described by Maurice[24] and by Dikstein and Maurice,[25] makes use of specular illumination to obtain an image of the corneal endothelial surface. Its coaxial illumination is through the objective lens that must be in contact with the corneal epithelium. This affords better resolution at ×500 magnification. In 1970, Hoefle et al.[26] modified the Maurice microscope by adding a holder to place eye bank eyes and enable them to be tilted in different directions so the whole corneal suface could be studied. For a better observation of the endothelium, Hoefle increased the intraocular pressure to 60 mm Hg by external compression. In this way, the postmortem corneal folds and corneal swelling decreased and allowed a clearer image of the endothelium. According to McCarey,[27] this examination can be done within 6 hr postmortem without the need for increasing the intraocular pressure. Eyes with extreme anisocytosis and cell population below 1000/sq mm are not acceptable donors by this method.

VITAL ENDOTHELIAL STAINING

Stocker,[28] in 1966, advocated the use of 0.25% trypan blue for the evaluation of corneal tissue just prior to keratoplasty. The excised donor cornea was put in a paraffin block with a well to hold it, and the cornea's concavity was filled with trypan blue. Several minutes later, the dye was removed, the cornea gently rinsed and examined under the microscope. This procedure could be done immediately before transplantation in the operating room, and the endothelium did not suffer with the application of this dye. In 1973, Van Horn[29] evaluated this method of estimating cell damage with the dye by using the electron microscope. Although this technique has not gained popularity, it really measures cell viability, and on this basis, Fernandez, Malbran, and Stefani[30] have screened over 180 corneas without a single case of primary tissue failure. These authors, however, used the mate cornea for keratoplasty. Lissamine green is another vital dye used by Hassard.[31] Its results are similar to those of trypan blue.

TEMPERATURE REVERSAL

Davson[32] and Harris and Nordquist[33] described the phenomenon known as "temperature reversal effect." When a fresh cornea is refrigerated, as in a moist chamber, the tissue swells but reverses to its precooling thickness after the cornea has been rewarmed to body temperature. Mishima and Kudo[34] showed that this effect is related to a decrease and recovery of active fluid transport by the endothelium into and out of the cornea. Hoefle[35] used this technique to test viability of cryopreserved corneas; and Sherrard[36] suggested using this technique for the evaluation of donor eyes and reported studies in animal eyes. He determined an ideal rate of reversal during a 2-hr period of incubation for tissue to qualify as excellent for penetrating keratoplasty.

The information obtained by experimental studies has served to correlate these findings in human eyes with other parameters of viability, i.e., age of the patient, time of death, time of enucleation, etc., nitro blue tetrazolium staining in some eyes, and histologic observations in others. All of this information can be summarized in a few statements: The younger the cornea, the better the donor tissue, the sooner the eye is removed after death, the better the tissue, and the same is true for the shorter period of time the eye remains on refrigeration. The use of the technique of short-term preservation immediately after enucleation has not only preserved the quality of normal endothelium, but extended its use to almost a whole week instead of 2 days, which was the maximum allowed by most surgeons.

NITRO BLUE TETRAZOLIUM STAINING

In 1964, Peña-Carrillo and I[37] described the use of nitro blue tetrazolium (NBT) salts to demonstrate the presence of lactic and succinic dehydrogenase enzymes in the stored corneal endothelium. We chose these enzymes after the demonstration by Berkow and Patz[38] and Baum[39] that their presence in the cornea indicated an active metabolic state. We also know that there are important elements in cellular metabolism, and some of these enzymes increase in cells injured by physical trauma. Our method required the incubation of fresh corneal tissue in the nitro blue tetrazolium media with a substrate (lactic or succinic dehydrogenases) for a period of time varying between 20 and 30 min until the formazan deposits were present in injured cells. Normal cells did not take up the stain, except for the intercellular junctions, which helped to differentiate the areas with and without cells or with destroyed endothelial cells. After 24 hr of storage, isolated areas of cell damage (staining) became confluent, forming large patches of endothelial cell damage. In another study, we attempted to correlate endothelial cell changes by the nitro blue tetrazolium technique in human eyes, and in the fellow eye we studied stromal oxygen consumption by the micropolarographic technique.[40] Biomicroscopic examination of these eyes showed no evidence of corneal disease, and in all cases, the biomicroscopic appearance of both eyes was similar. The period between death and enucleation was taken into account to compute the total storage time, which extended up to 264 hr. Fresh rabbit corneas incubated in the NBT media for demonstration of lactic dehydrogenases showed no staining; however, 10% of staining cells developed when rabbit corneas were stored for 26 hr. When the cornea was frozen and thawed before incubation, 100% of staining cells developed. With each cornea incubated, a fresh rabbit cornea was also incubated as a control. From our studies, we concluded that the *cadaveric time* (time between death and enucleation) must be added to the time of *eye bank storage* at 4°C. We introduced the concept of *total storage time* where consideration is given to this and the storage at 4°C. A short cadaveric storage time and a prolonged eye bank storage time may equate in endothelial changes to an eye that had several hours of cadaveric storage time and almost no eye bank storage time. We found that cadavers not maintained in a cold room, or with eyes partially open, would show endothelial cell changes. These studies correlated well with the observations on rabbit corneas, in that with prolonged storage in moist chambers, the NBT staining of endothelial cells also increased; but the staining was more extensive and pronounced in cells from eyes with prolonged cadaveric time. The stromal oxygen consumption of these corneas showed that as the cadaveric time and the storage time were prolonged, stromal respiration decreased and tissue thickness increased. It was also observed that human corneal stromal respiratory changes did not take place until after 24 hr (endothelial cell changes start much earlier). It seemed that the storage at 4°C prolonged the respiration of stromal cells, as previously found in rabbit corneas by Takahashi (personal communication). We also observed that corneal thickness measurement did not follow the drop in Q O_2 in endothelial duration. However, in practice, we like to obtain measurements of corneal thickness of donor eyes, since this is used as an additional parameter for the evaluation of corneal viability.

Another NBT staining method was described by Kaufman, Capella, and Robbins.[41] The technique indicated that the corneal tissue should be quickly frozen in order to rupture the cell membrane surface so the nitro blue tetrazolium should stain the cells. Nonstaining elements were considered dead, and the evaluation of the tissue was made on the basis of areas of no staining, whereas the previous technique counted the number of staining or injured cells. Both techniques have been extremely useful in the evaluation of corneal tissue for preservation, particularly at a time when cryopreservation was widely used, and one of the two corneas was used for endothelial study. Katowitz and Casey[42] also did an evaluation of experimental donor material with nitro blue tetrazolium staining. They reported a progressive increase of endothelial cell death after

+4°C storage in moist chambers or in the animal cadaver. The number of dead cells did not exceed 5% in corneas stored for 48 hr. They described the number of dead cells, while Peña and I described the number of injured cells or cells with a membrane more permeable to NBT salts. The method we used did not separate altered or injured cells from dead cells.

REFERENCES

1. Kaufman HE, Capella JA: Preserved corneal tissue for transplantation. J Cryosurg 1:125, 1968
2. Sakimoto T, Valenti J, Itai M, et al: Intermediate-term storage. Invest Ophthalmol 15:219, 1974
3. McCarey BE, Kaufman HE: Improved corneal storage. Invest Ophthalmol 13:165, 1974
4. Kuwahara Y, Sakanaue M: Studies on the long-term preservation of the cornea for penetrating keratoplasty. Acta Soc Ophthalmol Jap 69:1751, 1965
5. Mueller FO, Smith AU: Some experiments on grafting frozen corneal tissue in rabbits. Exp Eye Res 2:237, 1963
6. Bigar F, Kaufman HE, McCarey BE, et al: Improved corneal storage: Preliminary report on penetrating keratoplasties in humans. Am J Ophthalmol 79:115, 1975
7. Filatov VP: Optical transplantation of the cornea and tissue therapy. Moscow: State Publishers of Medical Literature. Excerpta Medica I. Ophthalmology. 57, 1947
8. Barraquer Moner JI: Safety techniques in penetrating keratoplasty. Trans Ophthalmol Soc UK 69:77, 1949
9. Katzin HM: The preservation of corneal tissue by freezing and dehydration. Am J Ophthalmol 30:1128, 1947b
10. Castroviejo R: Keratoplasty: Comments on the technique of corneal transplantation, source and preservation of donor's material. Report on new materials. Am J Ophthalmol 24:139, 1941
11. Thomas CI: Preservation of corneal tissue for transplantation. Arch Ophthalmol 36:321, 1946
12. Rollins HJ, Stocker FW: Bacterial flora and preoperative treatment of donor corneas. Am J Ophthalmol 59:247, 1965
13. Polack FM, Locatcher-Khorazo D, Gutierrez E: Bacteriologic study of donor eyes. Arch Ophthalmol 78:219, 1967
14. Doctor D, Hughes I: Prophylactic use of Neosporin for donor eyes. Am J Ophthalmol 46:351, 1958
15. Paton RT: Donor material, In: Keratoplasty. New York, McGraw-Hill, 1955
16. Bourne WM, McCarey BE, Kaufman HE: Clinical specular microscope. Trans Am Acad Ophthalmol Otolaryngol, 81:743, 1976
17. McCarey BE, Marshall W: Survey of eye banks and surgeons. Scientific Session E.B.A.A. Presentation, Dallas, 1975 (unpub)
18. De Roeth A Jr: Metabolism of the stored cornea. Arch Ophthalmol 44:659, 1950
19. King JH: Donor eyes and eye banks. Int Ophthalmol Clin 10:313, 1970
20. Stocker FW, King EH, Lucan DO, et al: Comparison of two different staining methods for evaluating cornea endothelial viability. Arch Ophthalmol 76:833, 1966
21. Schaeffer EM: Ultrastructural changes in moist chamber corneas. Invest Ophthalmol 2:272, 1963
22. Van Horn DL, Schultz RO: Ultrastructural changes in the endothelium of human corneas stored under eye bank conditions, In Capella JA, Edelhauser HF, Van Horn DL (eds): Corneal Preservation. Springfield, Ill, Charles C Thomas, 1973

23. Kalevar V: Donor corneas for keratoplasty. Tropical factors affecting its usability and viability. Br J Ophthalmol 49:491, 1965

24. Maurice DM: The location of the fluid pump in the cornea. J Physiol 221:43, 1972

25. Dikstein S, Maurice DM: The metabolic basis to the fluid pump in the cornea. J Physiol 221:29, 1972

26. Hoefle FB, Maurice DM, Sibley RC: Human corneal donor material: A method of examination before keratoplasty. Arch Ophthalmol 84:741, 1970

27. McCarey BE: Physiological evaluation of the corneal endothelium during and after cryopreservation. Ph.D. Dissertation, Marquette University, Milwaukee, June, 1972

28. Stocker FW: The endothelium of the cornea and its implications. Trans Am Ophthalmol Soc 56:669, 1954

29. Van Horn DL: Evaluation of trypan blue staining of the human corneal endothelim, In Capella JA, Edelhauser HF, Van Horn DL (eds): Corneal Preservation. Springfield, Ill, Charles C Thomas, 1973a

30. Fernandez Meijide RE, Malbran ES, Stefani C: Determinacion de la viabilidad endotelial en las queratoplastias perforantes. Arch Oftal B Aires 45, 1970

31. Jans RG, Hassard DTR: Lissamine green—A supravital stain for determination of corneal endothelial viability. Can J Ophthalmol 2:297, 1967

32. Davson H: The hydration of the cornea. Biochem J 59:24, 1955

33. Harris JE, Nordquist LT: The hydration of the cornea. I. The transport of water from the cornea. Am J Ophthalmol 40:100, 1955

34. Mishima S, Kudo T: In vitro incubation of rabbit cornea. Invest Ophthalmol 6:329, 1967

35. Hoefle FB: Human corneal donor material. In vitro studies. Arch Ophthalmol 32:361, 1969

36. Sherrard ES: Method of evaluating donor cornea for transplantation. Br J Ophthalmol 57:244, 1973a

37. Peña-Carrillo J, Polack FM: Histochemical changes in endothelium of corneas stored in moist chambers. Arch Ophthalmol 71:811, 1964

38. Berkow JW, Patz A: Histochemistry of Retina: I. Introduction and methods. Arch Ophthalmol 65:820, 1961

39. Baum JL: A histochemical study of corneal respiratory enzymes. Arch Ophthalmol 70:59, 1973

40. Polack FM, Kudo T, Takahashi GH: Viability of human eye bank cornea. Arch Ophthalmol 79:205, 1968

41. Kaufman HE, Capella JA, Robbins JE: Preservation of viable corneal tissue. Arch Ophthalmol 74:669, 1965

42. Katowitz JA, Casey TA: Endothelial viability of the rabbit cornea: A comparison of enucleated versus unenucleated forms of storage. In Puig-Solanes M (ed): International Congress of Ophthalmology, 21st. Mexico, 1970. Vol 1, Amsterdam 1971, Excerpta Medical Found

Part 2
Techniques and Instrumentation

Chapter 9

Microsurgical Instrumentation and Sutures

Surgery under the microscope is just one portion of the concept of microsurgical technique that must be applied to any field of ophthalmic surgery. In keratoplasty, these techniques acquire a most important place in our final results and possibly in reducing the incidence or severity of graft reactions (chapter 15). By performing surgery under the microscope, we learned to be more careful with the donor tissue, to improve our cuts or dissections, we designed finer instruments, and demanded better suture material and needles. We cannot attribute our improved results in keratoplasty to the use of the microscope alone, but to several surgical improvements, all of which depend on the surgeon's fine technique.

Magnifications larger than that afforded by surgical loupes was recommended by surgeons here and abroad in the early 1950s,[1-3] Perritt[1] being the first to use high magnification for anterior segment surgery in the United States before the microscope, as we know it, was designed (Fig. 9-1). It took almost 10 yr before the operating microscope, which was being used as culposcope or otoscope, was recognized as an indispensable instrument in eye surgery. Only in the late 1960s was it generally accepted in the U.S.A.

Because of these improvements, keratoplasty has progressed to the extent that it is now a rather frequent operation. We know more about corneal pathology than a few years ago, and we can predict which cases will have better keratoplasty results or why some cases fail.[2,3] Knowing the technical causes of failure also helps us to improve our technique or select our donor tissue better. We hope that this book will bring attention to the many factors, other than biologic problems, that play a role in the survival of a corneal graft. The surgeon should consider the microscope, instruments, and sutures only the tools to replace the cornea. The concept of microsurgery goes beyond the equipment.

THE MICROSCOPE

The use of the microscope must start years before a surgeon adopts it as a routine part of his equipment for corneal surgery. In most teaching institutions of the United States, residents start intraocular surgery with microscopic magnification; 2 or 3 yr later, the use of this instrument is part of their surgical setup and not an instrument that is an obstacle between their eyes and the patient. Hand–eye coordination under magnification needs a long period of time for precise and careful instrumentation, particularly when it is done under high

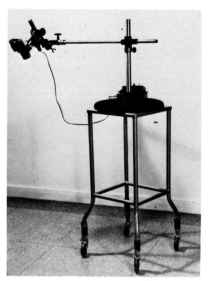

Figure 9-1.   Operating microscope used by R. A. Perritt in 1946 (courtesy of Dr. R. Perritt).

power. For this reason, it is advisable not to begin microsurgical corneal work with high magnification (×25 or more) if one has used this instrument only occasionally. A microscope affording ×8–×10 is satisfactory for the beginning microsurgeon. Another problem found by beginning microsurgeons is the fact that the operating microscope locks the surgeon in one spot. He can no longer move about the patient's head to place sutures in the eye with ease and comfort, but must learn to move both hands and fingers in ways never used before.[4] Some of the most difficult aspects are the placement of sutures with backstrokes or reverse motion and tying the sutures with fine instruments under the microscope.

Microscope objective lenses and eyepieces can vary in power; the focal length of the objective lens gives the working distance, and the combination of the two lenses with eyepieces gives the final magnification and the field of vision or "working field." The most comfortable working distance for corneal work is from 150 to 175 mm. Figure 9-2 shows the approximate working field for various magnifications. As one can see, at the magnification of ×40, the visual field is noticeably reduced.[5]

Light is provided by a coaxial system or lateral illumination (Fig. 9-3). Coaxial illumination is useful in anterior segment surgery when the red reflex of the retina is required to excise lens membranes, cortical material, or to remove vitreous.[5] For keratoplasty, however, the lateral illumination, as provided now by several scopes (Zeiss, Weck, Topcon, etc.), is better[6] because it reduces the glare and improves depth perception (Fig. 9-4). Most surgeons use both systems simultaneously.

Stability is another thing to look for in a microscope, since small vibrations are magnified, particularly over ×25. Most operating rooms are equipped with floor-stand models, but if possible, microscopes should be ceiling suspended.

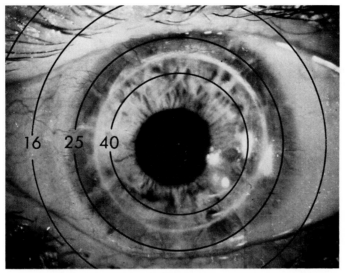

Figure 9-2. Operating field obtained with different microscopic magnifications.

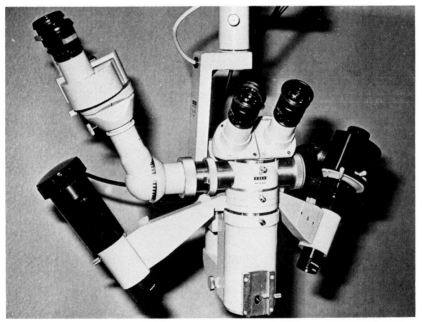

Figure 9-3. The Zeiss-Zoom microscope (OPMI–8) with coaxial and oblique illuminations, slit-lamp, and viewers scope.

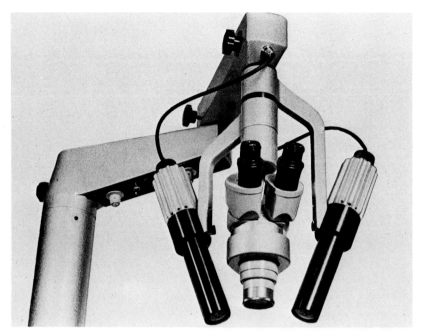

Figure 9-4. The Troutman-Weck microscope.

Most suspension systems work well, but vibration can still be transmitted if the operating room ceiling is not part of a firm construction.

Light weight or portable microscopes, such as the Codman-Mentor, Sparta, Alcon, Topcon, Olympus, etc., can be used for anterior segment surgery if magnification does not go over ×12. Since they are clamped to the surgical table or attached to a base, microscopes transmit vibrations that are acceptable at low magnifications. The Zeiss-Barraquer microscope is a small but very efficient instrument for anterior segment surgery. Because of its good optics, good focal depth, and lateral illumination it can satisfy most of the requirements for microsurgery. Motorized focusing and zoom optics are conveniences one may look for in one of the large microscopes, as well as assistant scope, slit lamp, etc. In some microscopes, these attachments increase excessively the body length and the distance eyepiece-objective.

A complement to the surgical microscope is a device to steady the hands, so the fine and controlled movements required during surgery can be reproduced through the procedure without fatigue. These devices are called arm rests and a variety of them are available as part of specially designed surgeon's chairs; unfortunately, these chairs are expensive and their arm rests do not always fit the operating table. Actually, most operating tables in the United States are not designed for eye surgery: the patient's head cannot be situated close enough to the surgeon; who has to lean forward away from his chair. We found that the best arm support under the circumstances is given by the "Chan arm rest" (Fig. 9-5). This device can be used as an extension of the operating table where an adjustable curved bar is located. The curved bar is positioned at the level of the patient's orbit.

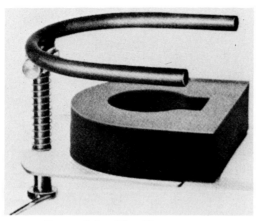

Figure 9-5. The Chan armrest.

INSTRUMENTS

Since the working distance between the patient's eye and the microscope objective lens is usually less than 200 mm, microsurgical instruments must be necessarily short to avoid touching the bottom of the microscope while operating. Size reduction, therefore, has been one of the modifications seen in microsurgical instruments as compared to old-fashioned instruments that were longer and heavier.[4] Finishing is more precise, particularly with needle holders and tying forceps, because these instruments must efficiently handle sutures as thin as 15 μ. Quality control for microsurgical instruments is usually good, but the surgeon must frequently check the instruments under the microscope to be sure that they have no flaws that may damage his suture material. A matte finish is also characteristic of microsurgical instruments to reduce the glare from the microscope lights.[6]

Microsurgical needle holders should handle only fine microsurgical needles; their jaws will be ruined if they are frequently used to drive large needles, therefore, for needles such as that attached to 4'0' and 5'0' silk, a larger needle holder should be used (Fig. 9-6). Reduction of tissue trauma is one of the principles of microsurgery, for this reason, corneal forceps should hold the corneal tissue without crushing. For corneal suturing, the following forceps are available: Bonn-Castroviejo (0.12 mm) forceps and the Barraquer colibri forceps (0.12) with rat teeth or with Pierse tips (Fig. 9-7). To handle scleral tissue we use the Castroviejo 0.3-mm forceps, which is an excellent instrument for general microsurgical use.[3] The McPherson, the Grieshaber Colibri (#696) or the jewelers forceps are ideal instruments for fine intraocular manipulation. As tying forceps, most frequently we use the Harms or the Paton forceps to handle nylon material. Other microsurgical forceps have been designed by Fine, Barraquer, Girard and Maumenee, and others.[7] The razor-blade knife is still the most useful and sharpest knife commonly available. Our preference is the Troutman right-angle razor-blade holder (Fig. 9-8). Perhaps equal sharpness can be obtained from a Diamond knife, but they are bulky and very expensive. "Beaver" makes very fine disposable microblades (no. 75), as does "Medical

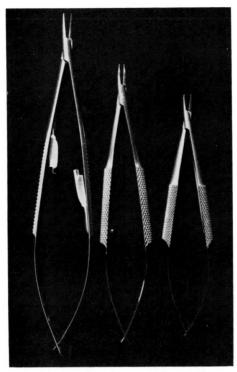

Figure 9-6. Castroviejo needleholder (left), Troutman microsurgical needleholder (center), Cohan microsurgical needleholder (right).

Workshop" (Holland) with their "superblade." Ultrasonically powered knives will eventually be used in anterior segment surgery, but one must remember that equally good results can be obtained with simple instruments. However, electromechanical knives are now being used.[8-10]

One of the causes of operative trauma to the graft is the excessive manipulation of the donor tissue when inserting the first suture. This was particularly critical with cryopreserved corneas, because their endothelial layer was more susceptible to trauma. In order to place the first suture in the graft, the transplant is often pressed against the recipient to avoid the rotation given when there is only one point of fixation. To prevent this problem, we designed a double-

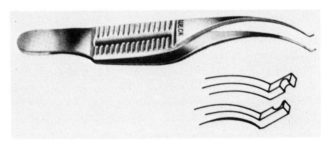

Figure 9-7. The Pierse microsurgical colibri forceps.

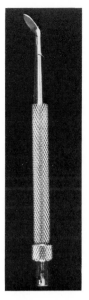

Figure 9-8. Angulated razor-blade knife (Troutman).

pronged tip on a colibri forceps (Fig. 9-9). The slit in the 0.12-mm toothed double forceps is only 1.5 mm in width, enough to let most microsurgical needles pass through.

Corneal scissors have been modified in size to conform to microsurgical techniques. We use the single curve Castroviejo scissors and the Troutman set. A perfect cut on the host cornea can be obtained with a mechanical trephine;[10] however, none of these instruments could make a complete through-and-through cut without risking iris or lens injury. A micrometric depth gauge is not essential in a trephine.[12] Many trephines are used today without such devices,

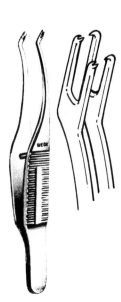

Figure 9-9. Double-pronged forceps for first suture in corneal graft (Polack).

which obliterate vision while cutting and increase the cost of the instrument. Final results, cosmetic and optical, do not seem to be undesirable if a trephine blade, knife, and scissors technique is used, as shown in chapter 11. I believe that this technique gives a controlled cut with an adequate beveling of the posterior half of the cornea.

Our preference is to use the Barraquer wire lid retractor and scleral support by means of Flieringa rings. We use them in phakic (single ring) and in aphakic eyes (double ring). Some of these rings have wings to hold the lids,[12-15] as shown in Figure 9-10.

NEEDLES AND SUTURE MATERIAL

The needles and sutures available today for microsurgical procedures are the response of industry to the demands of ophthalmic surgeons and to the generalized use of the operating microscope. It was only in the late 1950s, when fine ophthalmic needles were produced, that edge-to-edge suturing of corneal grafts became possible. The Vogt-Barraquer (Grieshaber 83) and Castroviejo (GR82) were the most famous needles before the swagged atraumatic needles were produced in the United States in 1959.[16] In contrast to eyed needles, which are commonly used in Europe, the swagged needles are almost exclusively used in the United States today. These needles are made of carbon or stainless steel, and both of these afford excellent sharpness for corneal surgery. The swagged needles have the obvious advantage of not requiring threading and being less traumatic since a single thread passes through the tissue, but this does not apply to monofilament nylon. Parallel to technology in manufacturing needles, technology also improved the textile industry so finer suture materials were available. When nylon sutures became available in 1960, a revolution occurred in corneal surgery, since up to that time only silk had been used.

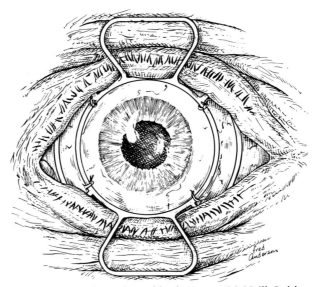

Figure 9-10.   Flieringa ring—blepharostat (McNeill-Goldman).

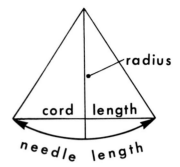

Figure 9-11. Diagram illustrating the various parameters to describe needle characteristics.

An ideal needle for anterior segment surgery should have the following characteristics:[17] (1) be sufficiently rigid so that curvature is not changed during passage; (2) be sufficiently long so that it can be grasped by the needle holder for passage through tissue and then be retrieved without damage to the point; (3) be of sufficient diameter (wire size) to afford a sharp point, cutting edge, and to make a tract large enough to allow retraction of the knot; and (4) be as atraumatic to the tissue as possible.

Needle description includes the following parameters: curvature, chord, radius, wire diameter, needle length, and shape (Fig. 9-11). The are usually made with three different curvatures: ½ circle, ⅜, and ¼ circle; and can also be described in degrees: 175°–180°, 130°–150°, and 90°–100° (Fig. 9-12). Half-circle needles are used for deep and short bites (deep-wound closure), whereas larger bites can be obtained with flatter needles, ⅜ and ¼ circle.

Atraumatic needles for corneal surgery are made of steel wire (stainless or carbon steel) and of diameters that vary from 0.15 mm to 0.23 mm. A cleft or an opening is made in the tail of the needle for manual insertion of the sutures,

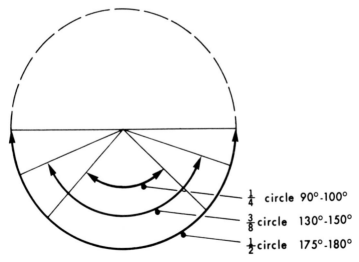

Figure 9-12. Diagram illustrating the various needle curvatures and their most common designations.

which are held in place by glue or closure of the cleft. The three basic body shapes of the needles are reverse cut, side cut, or spatulated and tapered (Fig. 9-13). In corneal surgery, the following makes of needles are used: spatula (Ethicon GS-8, 9, 10, 14), modified spatula (Davis and Geck LO-1), reverse cut (Davis and Geck CE-30).

The micropoint Ethicon needle is available in four curvatures, each curvature allowing a typical depth of insertion while maintaining the ends of the suture close to the wound (1.5 mm). Davis and Geck and Grieshaber needles are listed to the right.

GS-8 (97°)   Superficial placement (lamellar grafts) LO-1
GS-9 (135°) Medium depth (lamellar, penetrating) CE-30 GE-30
  (Grieshaber 82, 83)
GS-10 (175°) Deep insertion (penetrating) C-21
GS-14 (160°) Deep insertion (penetrating)

The round needle (BV-2 Ethicon with 10′ 0′ nylon) is ideal for iris suturing because it makes a perforation smaller than the wire used with the spatulated needles and 10′0′ material. These needles are used in microneurosurgery.

Silk (8′0′ and 9′0′) and nylon are two materials used in corneal surgery. Silk produces more reaction than nylon, and these characteristics can be used advantageously in edematous corneas, where some degree of reaction is required (see chapter 12). In the United States, we may obtain nylon material called "Perlon" or "Supramid." These are European names for nylon from a composition slightly different (Formula 6) from the nylon manufactured in the United States

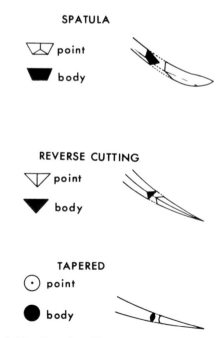

Figure 9-13. Drawing illustrating the various shapes of ophthalmic needles.

(Formula 6-6).[18] When a needle penetrates corneal tissue, it makes a perforation larger than the diameter of the suture material (Fig. 9-14). The 8'0' silk is the suture with a diameter more approximate to the diameter of the needle, and the same is true for 9'0' nylon. The difference in diameter between needle and suture makes it easier for the 10'0' nylon knotted suture to slide into the corneal perforation as is shown in Figure 9-15. This is not possible with 9'0' nylon or silk.

Davis and Geck (carbon steel) and Ethicon (stainless steel) needles, performed well without losing their sharpness after suturing one experimental graft (16–24 passages). Spatulated needles were easier to handle than reverse-cut needles for intralamellar work, especially for deep corneal wound closure or for lamellar keratoplasty. They stay in the planned tissue plane and follow the required curve. Needles with reverse cut (G-6, 8'0'; CE-30 8', 9'0') are preferred for penetrating tough tissue (dense corneal scarring, full-thickness scleral grafts, or full-thickness dehydrated corneas); they are preferred for through-and-through corneal sutures, showing greater facility in penetrating Descemet's membrane than spatulated needles, which showed a tendency to "skate" along it. This was also true in our clinical experience. Even though experimentally, silk and nylon sutures are covered by new Descemet's (Fig. 9-16), this technique of through-and-through suturing needs further investigation in humans. Blunt spatulated needles or improper technique may detach Descemet's membrane from the graft.

The disproportion between the needle diameter and the suture material is evident when we examined the tail of the GS-9 needles with 8'0' virgin silk (Fig. 9-17), 22-μ (Fig. 9-18), and 13-μ (Fig. 9-19) monofilament nylon attached. The

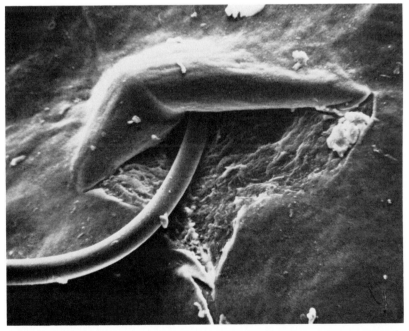

Figure 9-14. Scanning electron microphotograph showing the entrance point of a GS-9 needle with 9'0' monofilament nylon in a rabbit cornea (SEM, ×500).

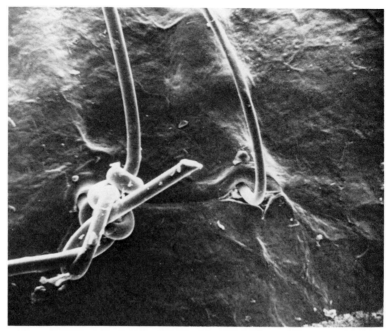

Figure 9-15. Electron microphotograph showing the relative size of 8′0′ and 9′0′ monofilament nylon sutures. The knot of the 10′0′ nylon suture (right); the knot of the 9′0′ sutures is too large to be run into the suture tract (SEM, ×200).

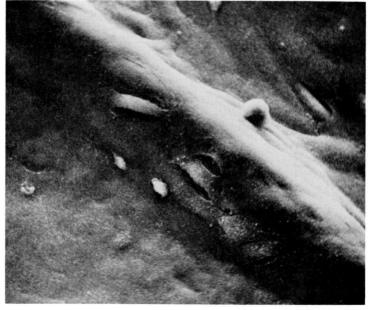

Figure 9-16. Scanning electron microphotograph of rabbit corneal endothelium covering a 10′0′ monofilament nylon suture placed through-and-through the cornea (SEM, ×500).

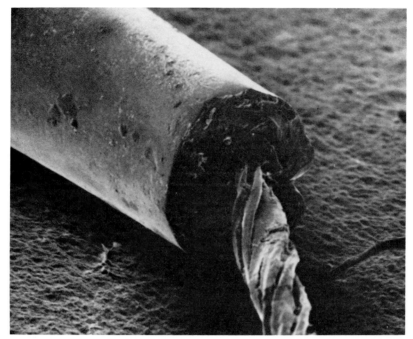

Figure 9-17. The tail of a microsurgical needle (GS-9) with 8′0′ virgin silk suture (SEM, ×200).

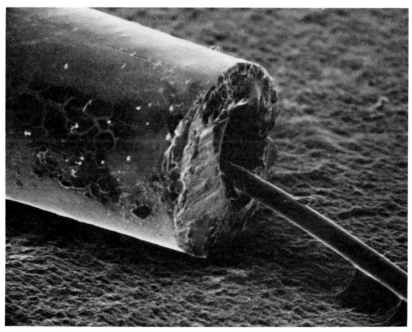

Figure 9-18. The tail of a GS-9 microsurgical needle with 10′0′ nylon suture material (SEM, ×200).

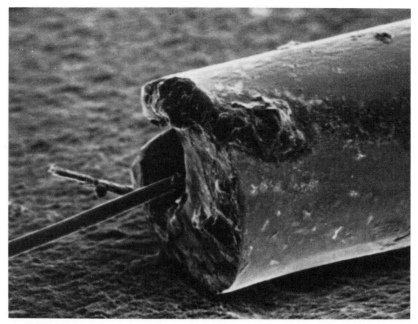

Figure 9-19. The tail of a GS-9 microsurgical needle with 13-μ nylon suture material (SEM, ×200).

shank opening for the suture insertion is too large for the monofilament material, and the edges of the openings too sharp. This accounts for the facility with which these sutures "break" when nylon is pulled against the edge of the shank. The suture is cut, not broken.

CONTROL OF LINT AND DEBRIS IN THE OPERATIVE FIELD

Even though a discussion of this sort does not really belong in a chapter on microsurgery, it probably has a place here because in our concept of microsurgery we encompass all aspects of ocular surgery, including any process that may induce tissue reaction and interfere with our desired results. Cotton drapes and gowns are some of the worst offenders in intraocular surgery because of the large amount of lint they produce. Lint is probably one of the frequent causes of inflammatory reactions after surgery that has been ignored in the past. The use of special plasticized paper for gowns and drapes has decreased this problem, which was most noticeable in lamellar keratoplasties. Powdered gloves are now routinely eliminated in eye surgery, as are cotton applicators, and solutions for intraocular use are now passed through Millipore filters to eliminate foreign particles. The set-up shown in Figure 9-20 is one which, in our experience, has been quite satisfactory to control the problem of lint produced by gowns and drapes. Once intraocular surgery has started, it is

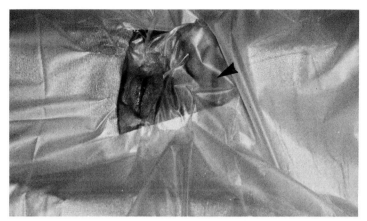

Figure 9-20. Plastic-coated drapes to eliminate lint in the operating field. A small plastic eye drape will cover the operating area. Arrow indicates airway under drapes.

advisable to eliminate unnecessary traffic in the operating room, since personnel or visitors circulating around the floor may still produce enough lint or particulate matter to defeat the purpose of the plasticized drapes.

REFERENCES

1. Perritt RA: Micro-ophthalmic surgery. Proceedings of the XX International Congress of Ophthalmology, Munich, 1966, p 912, Weigelin E, (ed.) Excerpta Medica Found. 1967
2. Barraquer J, Rutllan J: Surgery of the Anterior Segment of the Eye, vol II, Corneal Surgery. Barcelona, Institute Barraquer, 1971
3. Castroviejo R: Atlas de Queratomias y Queratoplastias, Barcelona, Salvat, 1964
4. Troutman R: Microsurgery of the Anterior Segment of the Eye. St. Louis, C.V. Mosby, 1974
5. Roper-Hall MJ: The development and application of microsurgery. Trans Ophthalmol Soc (Eng) 87:195, 1967
6. Harms H, Mackensen G: Ocular Surgery Under the Microscope. Chicago, Yearbook Medical, 1967
7. Paton D: Penetrating keratoplasty: Advocation of microscopic management and an arbitrary selection of incision and suturing techniques. Highl Ophthalmol 13:213, 1970–1971
8. Pierse D: Alpha-chymnotrypsin in cataract surgery. Trans Ophthalmol Soc UK 80:423, 1960
9. Pericic L, Crock G, Heinze J: Vibrating microsurgical sectioning. Br J Ophthalmol 57:425, 1973
10. Nursall JF: A vibrating knife for ocular surgery. Trans Am Acad Ophthalmol 79:425, 1975
11. Draeger J: Newe Schneidetechnik in der Mikrochirurgie. Klin Monatsbl Augenheilkd 161:193, 1972

12. Naumann G: Einfachedr Keratoplastik-trepan zur Verwendung unter dem Operations-mikroskop. Klin Monatsbl Augenheilkd 161:708, 1972

13. Mackensen G: Eine modifikation des Flieringaschrz skleralringes. Klin Monatsbl Augenheilkd 148:280, 1966

14. Madroszkiewicz M: Ein Selbsttragender palpebroskleraler ring sog. Henkel-Ring zur Verhütung des Glaskorpervorfalls. Klin Monatsbl Augenheilkd 161:707, 1972

15. McNeill J, Goldman K, Kaufman HE: Combined scleral ring and blepharostat. Am J Ophthalmol 83:592, 1977

16. Rizutti AB: Clinical Evaluation of Suture Material and Needles in Surgery of the Cornea and Lens. A. B. Rizutti (pub) 1968 (Brochure) Ethicon, Inc., Somerville, N.J.

17. Polack FM, Sanchez J, Eve R: Microsurgical sutures: I. Evaluation of various types of needles and sutures for anterior segment surgery. Can J Ophthalmol 9:42, 1974

18. McPherson SD, Crawford J: The use of nylon sutures in anterior segment surgery. Eye Ear Nose Throat Mon 49:420, 1970

Chapter 10

Nonpenetrating (Lamellar) Keratoplasty

Transplantation of a portion of the stromal thickness was performed by Von Hippel in 1888, and in contrast to penetrating keratoplasty, this method of grafting became the operation of choice in Europe for many years. Today, we know that diseases affecting the deep stromal layers or Descemet's membrane and its endothelium will require a full-thickness keratoplasty. One advantage of partial-thickness, or lamellar, keratoplasty is that it can be performed with non-viable corneas. This is of valuable service in areas where fresh or preserved tissue is unavailable. A properly done lamellar graft requires expertise and good instrumentation. The results then are rewarding when this procedure is indicated, and all diseased tissue has been removed from the recipient cornea. Visual acuity seldom reaches the 20/20 level, but in most cases, a vision between 20/40 and 20/30 can be obtained. Today, with the aid of the microscope, we can perform a pre-Descemet's keratoplasty,[1] which can give the best visual results, providing that the endothelial layer is normal. Complications of lamellar keratoplasty are rare, and if results are not satisfactory, the graft can be repeated or a penetrating keratoplasty can be performed.

INDICATIONS

Lamellar keratoplasty is indicated for optical and for tectonic purposes. In diseases or dystrophies of the anterior corneal layers (Bowen's disease, Reiss-Buckler's dystrophy), a thin keratectomy is usually enough (Fig. 10-1**A–G**). However, if more than one-third of the corneal thickness has to be excised, it is convenient to place a thin lamellar graft.

Lamellar keratoplasty is contraindicated in corneal edema, severe corneal vascularization, and active stromal infection.

Optical Keratoplasties

1. Dystrophies and degenerations of the anterior corneal layers, when a keratectomy would not remove all superficial scar tissue; recurrent Reiss-Buckler's dystrophy; Saltzmann Nodular Degeneration
2. Dystrophies and degenerations of the corneal stroma, not compromising the deeper stromal layers; superficial granular dystrophy; crystalline dystrophy of Schneider
3. Traumatic or infectious leukomas

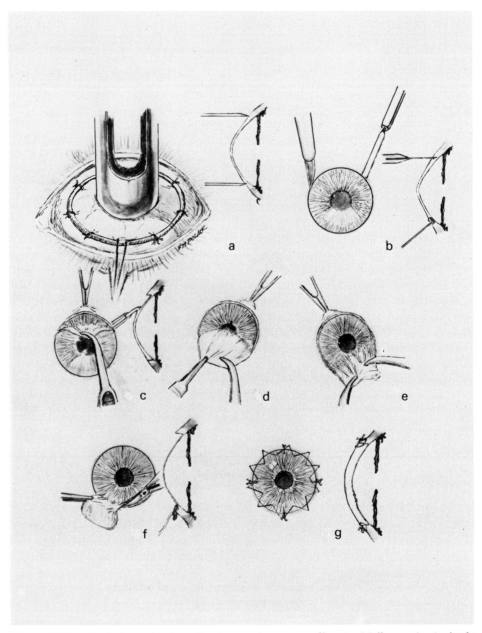

Figure 10-1. Technique for lamellar keratoplasty according to Malbran. **A.** A single Flieringa ring is in place; superficial trephination has been made with a 9.5-mm trephine. **B.** The cut is deepened with a razor-blade knife, and the edges of the corneal button are lifted with a Paufique knife 360°. **C.** The corneal tissue is pulled off with slow traction. **D.** Two forceps are used to pull the cornea over the corneal apex. **E.** The tissue is pulled down. **F.** The tissue is excised with scissors. **G.** The graft is secured with interrupted or running sutures.

4. Superficial burns with mild to moderate superficial vascularization (heavy or deep vascularization has a bad prognosis for lamellar keratoplasty)
5. Keratoconus and keratoglobus without previous breaks in Descemet's membrane
6. Postherpetic recurrent erosion, (metaherpetic keratopathy)

Therapeutic Keratoplasty (Tectonic Lamellar)

1. Corneal thinning (secondary to keratoconus, collagen diseases, etc.)
2. Stromal herpetic keratitis, ulcerated with mild vascularization; postherpetic keratopathy
3. Descemetocele
4. Marginal ulcerations
5. Pterygium (recidivant)
6. Dermoids and carcinomas of the limbus
7. Recurrent erosion with superficial scarring
8. Total corneal necrosis

INSTRUMENTS

Lid speculum (Barraquer wire speculum), trephine (disposable Weck trephine blade), Flieringa ring (Single ring, medium and large sizes)
Troutman-Llobera ring forceps
Lamellar dissectors
Paufique knife
Beaver #66 blade
Castroviejo curved scissors
Needle holder
5'0' dacron sutures (to secure ring)
8'0' silk or 10'0' nylon suture material
Suture scissors
Tissue forceps
Harms or Paton tying forceps
Bonn (0.12) or Pierse tissue forceps

SURGICAL TECHNIQUE

Akinesia of the lids is performed by a Van Lint method, using 2% Xylocaine with adrenalin (8–10 cc). Retrobulbar anesthesia is also done with 2% Xylocaine. In reoperations, we add 10,000 U of hyaluronidase.

After inserting the lid speculum, a single Flieringa ring, is secured to the episcleral tissue 5–7 mm behind the limbus with six 5'0' dacron sutures, as shown in Figure 10-1**A**. The purpose of this ring is to stabilize the eye and replace the usual superior and inferior rectus fixation with a more solid and regular support. In addition, the ring will avoid the deformation of the globe and will favor fixation with the special ring forceps at the time of corneal trephination or lamellar dissection. The four long sutures that hold the ring are secured to the drapes with mosquito clamps, and at the same time, the ring and the cornea are positioned parallel to the microscope objective lens. With few exceptions, we aim for a deep[9] lamellar keratoplasty, and our preferences are diameters of 7.5 mm or larger. The disposable Weck trephine blade is lightly stained with methylene blue on its cutting edge, and under direct microscopic visualization, the blade is centered on the cornea (the ring being held parallel to the microscope with the ring forceps). The trephine is then lightly rotated on the corneal surface until a superficial corneal cut is made. A slight tilting of the trephine edge will allow the surgeon to examine the depth of the cut. If the cut is not deep enough, another rotation of the trephine will penetrate the cut slightly deeper. The methylene blue will facilitate the determination of the depth of the cut. This superficial cut with the trephine is deepened with a razor-blade knife, as shown in Figure 10-1 **B**, until one estimates that deeper layers of the cornea have been reached by frequently lifting the graft with a fine forceps. This deepening cut with the razor-blade knife is continued around the 360° circumference, and then a cleavage plane is obtained in one of the quadrants with a Paufique knife. With this knife, one may lift the edge of the corneal tissue to be excised, and dissection can be continued around the edge of the corneal button with a Beaver #66 blade. Once we have reached this stage, there are two techniques to follow.

1. *Malbran's technique* is most useful for cases of keratoconus, keratoglobus, or very thin corneas without scarring. It is also called the "peeling off" technique, and consists of holding the edge of the cornea to be resected with two heavy forceps, and while the assistant holds the ring, the surgeon pulls the diseased corneal tissue downwards until most of the tissue has been removed from the deeper layers. The tissue excision is completed with scissors (Fig. 10-1 **C–F**).

2. *Technique with lamellar dissectors*[1-5] is usually done in situations where scar tissue in the stroma prevents the use of the previous technique. A combination of the two techniques is useful in some instances where the amount of scar tissue is small and localized to one area of the cornea. In some cases, the dissection of the corneal tissue can be effected with curved corneal scissors as done by Castroviejo.

As soon as the corneal tissue has been excised, it should be placed again on its previous bed, until the graft is ready to be sutured. Failure to do this will allow lint or floating debris to be deposited on the corneal surface, which will become apparent at the graft interface only after the graft has healed. The donor tissue must be of full thickness (minus Descemet's membrane), and placed on the patient's eye immediately after removing the diseased cornea (cotton swabs should be avoided during this procedure). The corneal graft is usually of similar size as the excised cornea, and therefore, at the time of suturing, it is necessary to do a small paracentesis in order to fit the graft properly on its bed. This paracentesis is done at the corneal limbus with a Wheeler knife or with the razor-blade knife, as shown in Figure 10-1 **G**. Four cardinal sutures are usually placed with 8'0' black silk, which are left in place until the 10'0' running nylon suture is completed. In selective cases, we may choose to use 8'0' virgin silk in an interrupted fashion, because healing will occur much faster with this material, and sutures can be removed within 4–6 wk, in contrast to the nylon material, which will require 3–4 mo before its removal.

After the Flieringa ring is removed, 10 mg of a soluble steroid is injected subconjunctivally (Dexamethasone), and an antibiotic ointment is applied to the corneal surface.

Obtaining the Graft

There are many ways to cut a lamellar graft from a whole donor eye. We have mentioned before that eyes for lamellar keratoplasty can be preserved at +4°C for about 1 wk, or kept frozen in liquid nitrogen, carbon dioxide, or in an electric freezer at low temperatures, (−79° to −150°). The loosened corneal epithelium of the thawed eye is removed with gauze, and the surface of the cornea is treated with antibiotic drops. Some surgeons prefer corneas less than 24 hours old.[11] These we use in keratoconus cases.

GRAFT REMOVAL WITH DISSECTORS

There are two techniques available. (1) Deep corneal lamellar dissection started from the limbus[2,3,6,12] (Fig. 10-2) after either a scratch incision or cut with a portion of a calibrated trephine set at a depth of 0.6 mm or less. A dissector is introduced through this cut with a push, and with right-and-left motion, the anterior corneal layers are dissected. Dissectors with serrated borders (Troutman) are best for this procedure. The graft of desired size is now cut from the central cornea. (2) The graft is cut first and then dissected. Dissection of the graft is started with a Paufique knife in one quadrant so a longer dissector may be used (Troutman's dissectors, Beaver blade #66, or the dull side of a razor-blade knife). Once a cleavage plane has been found, it must be followed uniformly. The dissectors are moved from side to side, while the tissue is gently lifted and

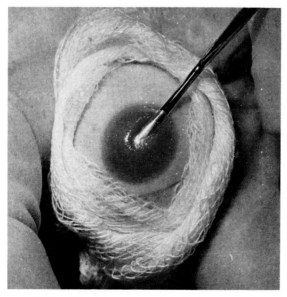

Figure 10-2. Obtaining a partial-thickness graft with a corneal dissector.

pulled. Care must be taken not to damage the edges of the graft with this maneuver. The cut at the edges is completed with curved scissors. Another method of dissecting the graft is by using curved corneal scissors, as described by Castroviejo[2] (Fig. 10-3). Once cut, the graft is immediately placed on the recipient bed.

GRAFT REMOVAL WITH ELECTRIC KERATOME

This instrument (Fig. 10-4) gives excellent grafts up to 8 mm if properly used. If one desires to obtain a graft 0.4-mm thick, a gauge 0.6-mm must be used if the cornea of the eye is edematous (an increase of 0.1 is also recommended for grafts obtained by the two previous methods). The cut is made in the cornea after epithelium removal with gauze and after a small trench has been made at the host edge on the corneal limbus. To engage the keratome, about normal intraocular pressure is given to the donor eye with the left hand, while the keratome is applied to the cornea with uniform pressure and while it is advanced following the corneal curvature.

FULL STROMAL THICKNESS GRAFTS

These are obtained from donor eyes or excised glycerol-preserved corneas. Once the graft is cut to the desired size, Descemet's membrane is removed with a blade and scissors under the operating microscope. These grafts are used for deep lamellar resections for the pre-Descemet keratoplasty.[9,10] Partial-thickness grafts from excised corneas (dehydrated) or corneas preserved in M-K media, require the use of the Furness clamp or a similar fixation device. The dissection of the graft is then performed as method 1. A service provided by some eye banks is that of preserving large precut grafts of 1 or 2 thicknesses (i.e., 0.3 and

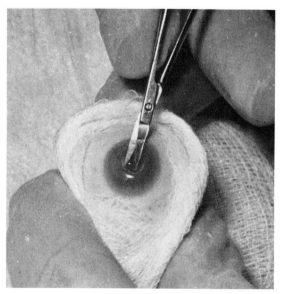

Figure 10-3. Curved corneal scissors used to dissect a laminar corneal graft.

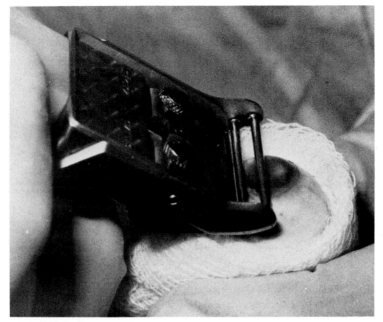

Figure 10-4. Castroviejo electric keratome in use. A small trench is made near the limbus to engage the blade.

0.4) in glycerol or in silica gel. These grafts can be readily rehydrated and cut to smaller sizes.

In most instances we use thick lamellar grafts (0.4 mm or more); obviously, these grafts are thicker when obtained from an edematous cornea, and allowance is made for tissue dehydration. Even though grafts cut with the electric keratome tend to give more myopia than grafts dissected with spatulas, they have a more uniform base, and the host–donor plane heals so well that the junction is unnoticeable.

COMPLICATIONS DURING SURGERY

Perforation of the Anterior Chamber While Deepening the Trephine Cut

This complication is immediately detected by the release of aqueous humor, and should this occur, the knife dissection in this area is discontinued and started in a different place. If the perforation at the edge of the cut is larger than 1 mm, it may require a transitory suturing of the whole cornea with 8'0' silk material. Careful dissection of the corneal tissue with instruments may have to start from the opposite area to the perforation, which now will be slightly more difficult if the eye has been made softer by the release of aqueous humor. Perforation of the host-lamellar bed after the corneal tissue has been partially excised may be corrected by suturing this rupture with 10'0' monofilament nylon if the break is not in the optical axis. If the break is central, or if it is too large or impossible to close with 10′0′ nylon, it will be necessary to convert this procedure to that of a penetrating keratoplasty. Attempts to cover a break of the lamellar bed with a corneal graft will usually end in the formation of a pseudochamber and opacification of the lamellar graft.

Bleeding Into the Lamellar Bed

Usually, blood retained between the graft and the lamellar bed is reabsorbed; however, in many instances a discoloration of this interface may occur with posterior deposition of lipid material. It is wise, therefore, to rinse the blood from the corneal surface before the graft is sutured. Should bleeding occur at the time of graft suturing, every effort should be made not to lift the graft from the bed so blood will not seep under its surface. To some extent, this complication can be prevented by the instillation of a solution of diluted adrenalin into the trephine cut before complete excision of the corneal tissue (adrenalin 1:20,000).

Inability to Approximate Wound Edges

This can be corrected or prevented by making the eye softer with the release of additional aqueous humor from the paracentesis incision.

Sutures Will Not Hold on Soft or Necrotic Host Tissue

In this situation, it is not recommended to use a running suture, use 8′0′ silk material in an interrupted fashion. Large bites in host tissue should prevent this material from cutting through the soft cornea. In the graft, the sutures should be placed through the whole thickness of the tissue. In areas of vascularization, 10′0′ nylon material is a better choice, but can be alternated with interrupted 8′0′ silk material.

POSTOPERATIVE COMPLICATIONS

Vascularization of the Graft

This usually develops in host corneas that have been heavily vascularized. In this type of host cornea, vascularization usually invades the host–graft interface, a situation that is most difficult to correct and a potential problem for future keratoplasty. Intensive steroid therapy and early suture removal may delay or stop this type of vascularization. The best treatment of this complication is its prevention. It has been mentioned before that lamellar grafts are not indicated in corneas with vascularization due to interstitial keratitis, herpetic keratitis, and chemical burns. Superficial vascularization usually disappears after suture removal or with steroid therapy.

Wound Dehiscence

If resuturing of the wound is not possible because of necrosis of the wound edges, it is convenient to apply a large (13.5 mm) soft contact lens. These lenses will prevent the development of edema of the graft borders with its consequent melting and progressive separation from the host edge.

Epithelial Defects

Many of the conditions for which lamellar keratoplasty are performed are associated with decreased tear production. Lamellar keratoplasty may aggravate this situation, and ulcerations of the graft's surface may end with stromal scarring (and even perforation). This situation should be immediately treated with a bandage soft contact lens, or if the ulceration is involving only the epithelium, it can be managed with frequent use of artificial tears and ointments during the day and ointment at bedtime. Evaluation of the tear function and lid closure prior to surgery should prevent this type of complication.

Infection of the Graft

It is not unusual to observe small suture abscesses in corneal transplants, however, in most instances, these are aseptic areas of necrosis around the suture. These tiny suture abscesses are more frequently observed around silk material, but can occur with interrupted or running nylon sutures. Should a true abscess be observed around the suture material, the suture should be removed and placed in an agar plate for culture and future investigation of the type of bacteria. Infections in the bed of the graft, or graft interface, usually occur at the time of surgery and are often related to the presence of foreign bodies at this level. We have observed gram-positive abscesses as well as fungal infections at the graft interface, and this type of disease will require immediate removal of the graft and treatment of the open graft interface until the infection appears to be controlled.

Epithelial Ingrowth

This complication may be evident shortly after keratoplasty, and it is manifested by a cloudy film or spots under the graft. It is due to a small separation of the wound, loose sutures, uneven graft or host border, small graft, or increased intraocular pressure. Fortunately, it is very rare, but if it keeps progressing, a penetrating graft will be necessary.

Graft Edema

According to Castroviejo, the early postoperative graft edema is due to a perforation of the host cornea. If the break is small, it will seal and the graft will clear; but if it is large, a pseudochamber will develop. In this case, a penetrating graft will be indicated.

Foreign Bodies in the Graft Bed

This complication can be minimized by not using cotton sponges in the field and by keeping the host cornea covered at all times after completing the keratectomy. The host cornea is uncovered only to place the graft. Cellulose sponges can also leave small foreign bodies. Sometimes these may cause inflammatory reactions that may simulate a fungal abscess.

Graft Rejection

Immune reactions are likely to occur in large (9–11 mm) lamellar grafts, usually 4–6 wk after keratoplasty. Edema of the graft with cloudiness and vascularization are signs of rejection. Sutures (if interrupted) must be removed, at least in alternate days, while topical and systemic steroids are used. After the rejection episode, if the graft has cleared, we like the patient to continue using daily steroid drops for several (8–10) months. In cases of large grafts, one drop a day of 0.1% Dexamethasone is used after surgery for approximately 1 yr. According to Fine,[10] the incidence of rejection of lamellar grafts is between 4% and 5%.

ATYPICAL LAMELLAR GRAFT

Sometimes the location or extension of the corneal pathology requires a corneal graft of unusual shape. A key-hole graft, for example, is performed when the central portion of the cornea requires lamellar grafting as well as a peripheral portion, as in pterygium. Instead of performing a total lamellar graft, which has a possibility of rejection, a choice is to remove only the central portion that is opaque and the segmental peripheral area with some overlapping of the graft on the scleral tissue. The anular lamellar graft is usually done for marginal degenerations or ectasias of the cornea comprising almost 360°. In other cases of marginal corneal degenerations or paracentral lesions, we may use rectangular, square, oval, segmental, or sectorial grafts.[4-7] Segmental grafts may have a straight, convex, or concave border. These three types of borders are used to minimize the amount of donor tissue grafted, while at the same time, all the diseased tissue is removed and a minimal amount of normal tissue is disrupted. Curved borders are easier to fit, since they are cut with trephines, (usually in diameters of 10 or 11 mm). The straight-top segmental graft is cut freehand and requires some expertise. A perfect scleral bed is not necessary as long as the graft is thin. The tissue can be sutured over the sclera and covered with conjunctiva. Rectangular or square grafts are also difficult to cut, unless one uses the double knife of Castroviejo or Pierse's razor-blade knife with guide.[8]

REFERENCES

1. Paufique L, Charleux J: Lamellar keratoplasty, *In* Casey TA (ed): Corneal Grafting. London, Butterworths, 1972, pp 121–176
2. Castroviejo R: Queratoplastia Lamelar, Atlas de Queratectomias y Queratoplastias. Barcelona, Salvat, 1964, pp 77-100
3. Offret G, Pouliquen Y: La greffe lamellaire, *In*: Les Greffes de la Corneé. Paris, Masson et Cie, 1974
4. Paton RT, Smith B, Katzin HM: Atlas of Eye Surgery. New York, McGraw-Hill, 1962
5. Harms H, Mackensen G: Ocular Surgery Under the Microscope. Chicago, Yearbook Medical, 1967
6. Troutman R: Microsurgery of the Anterior Segment of the Eye. St. Louis, C.V. Mosby, 1974
7. Barraquer J, Ruttllan J: Surgery of the Anterior Segment of the Eye, vol II. Corneal Surgery. Barcelona, Institute Barraquer, 1971
8. Pierse D, Eustace P: Instruments, *In* Casey TA (ed): Corneal Grafting, London, Butterworths, 1972, p 281
9. Vasco-Posada J: Homoqueratoplastia interlaminar. Rev Soc Col Oftal 4:99, 1973
10. Fine M: Lamellar corneal transplantation, *In*: Dabezies OH, Gitter KA, Samson CLM (eds): Symposium on the Cornea. Transactions of the New Orleans Academy of Ophthalmology. St. Louis, C.V. Mosby, 1972, p 204
11. Rocha H: Lamellar keratoplasty, Rev Bras Oftalmol 12:51, 1953
12. Galvao PG: Transplante de Cornea. Thesis faculdade de medicina da Univ. Fed. minas Gerais, Belo Horizonte, Brazil, 1976

Chapter 11

Penetrating Keratoplasty

Full-thickness corneal transplantation is indicated in patients with deep stromal opacities that cannot be removed by lamellar keratoplasty and alterations of Descemet's membrane (congenital dystrophies, fibrous membranes, Fuchs' dystrophy, etc.). In many cases, midstromal opacities of inflammatory origin have associated changes in Descemet's membrane and the endothelium (endothelial fibrous plaque) that require penetrating grafts if visual acuity must be corrected to normal. Decreased visual acuity to levels below 20/100 is only one of the parameters used to judge the indication for this type of corneal surgery. Once we have eliminated the possibility of decreased vision due to alterations of the lens and vitreous or macular alterations, a refraction with a contact lens may give us the best obtainable visual acuity. Often, the decreased visual acuity is due not so much to existing corneal opacities, but the irregular surface of the cornea. In previous chapters, we have seen that even if corneal grafting has a high success rate, results are by no means predictable, and the advantages and disadvantages of the surgery must be carefully considered and discussed with the patient, particularly the binocular patient with good vision in one eye and severe anterior segment alterations in the other. A cosmetic shell would be a good alternative in this case. Even if there is an indication for surgery, one should seriously consider the need for penetrating keratoplasty in the aged patient with 20/100 vision or less due to nonprogressing corneal disease, because they may have to be subjected to hyperosmotic agents, carbonic anhydrase inhibitors, and systemic steroids with their well known side effects. Most ophthalmologists are aware of the indications for penetrating keratoplasty, but not all are aware of the contraindications or how important it is to look for conditions that may cause graft failure. However, even if some conditions prevent surgery (acute inflammation), most of them can be modified or controlled; we refer to these as relative contraindications.

RELATIVE CONTRAINDICATIONS FOR PENETRATING KERATOPLASTY

Glaucoma

Often listed in many textbooks as an absolute contraindication, glaucoma is often undetected in keratoplasty because most optical and mechanical tonometers do not register the correct intraocular pressure in abnormal corneas. Determination of the intraocular pressure is part of the complete eye examination preceding keratoplasty. Two instruments give adequate pressure readings in corneas with irregular surfaces: the electronic tonometers (MacKay-Marg) and the air tonometers (Applamatic, Block Engineering, Mass.; Alcon Pneumotonograph, Texas) (Figs. 11-1 and 11-2). Pressures above normal must be reduced with miotics or carbonic anhydrase inhibitors, particularly if the eye is aphakic, because they tend to develop higher intraocular pressures after surgery.[1]

Eyes with elevated pressures that cannot be controlled with medical therapy may require filtering operation or cyclocryotherapy before keratoplasty. In exceptional cases, one may consider filtering surgery (sclerectomy under scleral flap) at the time of keratoplasty. Following cyclocryotherapy, one must wait for the intraocular inflammation to subside, even if the intraocular pressure has been normalized. After filtering surgery, we usually wait 2 mo before performing keratoplasty.

Dry Eye (Sjögren's Syndrome, Stevens-Johnson Syndrome)

It is important to reduce the inflammatory process in these eyes prior to surgery by fitting them with soft contact lenses (if the degree of dryness is not excessive) and prescribing frequent use of normal saline solution drops.[2] In addition, these patients must be given topical antibiotics (Gentamicin, Chloromycetin), and they should have lid margin scrubs with nonirritating baby soap, because they often have associated staphylococcal blepharitis.

At the end of the surgical procedure, the eye should be fitted again with a soft contact lens and continue with the frequent instillation of saline drops. Incomplete lid closure, trichiasis, entropion, lagophthalmos, etc. are some condi-

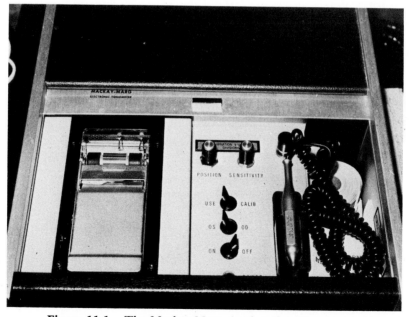

Figure 11-1. The Mackay-Marg Applanation Tonometer

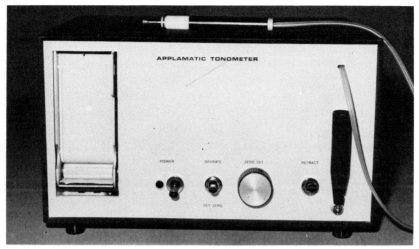

Figure 11-2.   The Air Tonometer (Applamatic) manufactured by Block Engineering

tions that must be corrected to prevent graft damage and eventual failure.[3] They are discussed in chapter 16.

Corneal Anesthesia

Corneal anesthesia due to herpes zoster or surgical neurectomy has been considered another contraindication for keratoplasty. In the past, these grafts did not heal well, the epithelium tended to slough, and they eventually opacified. The protection afforded by bandage soft contact lenses has modified the prognosis in these cases, provided the lenses are placed immediately after surgery, and the eye has adequate tear production or the lens is kept wet with saline solution.

Extreme Corneal Thinning in Keratoconus and Keratoglobus

Host corneas with thicknesses of less than 0.3 mm are high risk for complications in penetrating keratoplasty (graft ectasia, poor healing, retrograft membrane, iris adhesion). For this reason, I feel that a tectonic lamellar graft is indicated as preparatory for full-thickness keratoplasty.[4] Sometimes, the vision obtained is better than 20/40 with the lamellar graft.

Keratoplasty in Acute Hydrops

Some surgeons do not hesitate to perform a penetrating keratoplasty during the stage of acute corneal edema in keratoconus. Basically, this is not a contraindication, but I feel that it is better to wait for the resolution of the edema for two reasons: (1) visual acuity sometimes improves after edema subsides, and (2) healing is inadequate in edematous corneas due to diminution in the number of keratocytes. Also, a better tissue thickness match may be obtained after the edema has resolved.

Herpetic Keratitis

We like to wait for a period of inactivity of several months (6–10 mo) duration before penetrating keratoplasty. This subject is discussed more extensively in chapter 15.

Trauma

In cases of trauma, there are no fixed guidelines about indications or contraindications for full-thickness keratoplasty. If the amount of corneal damage is extensive in a perforating injury, we feel that it is best to do all anterior chamber repair during the initial surgery and replace the damaged cornea with a corneal graft.[5]

INSTRUMENTS NECESSARY FOR PENETRATING KERATOPLASTY

Lid speculum (Barraquer wire speculum)

Fixation forceps (0.5-mm teeth)

Flieringa rings (12 through 22 mm), single rings for phakic eyes and double rings for aphakic eyes (small and large size)

Razor-blade holder (Troutman, angled)

Forceps: Troutman-Llobera ring forceps, Bonn forceps (0.12), Colibri Pierse (0.12), Jeweler's forceps, Polack (Weck) double corneal graft forceps

Scissors: Vannas, Castroviejo single curve, Troutman-Castroviejo right and left, corneal graft scissors, Westcott sharp and blunt scissors.

Iris spatula, Paton spatula, Barraquer vitreous spatula

Wheeler knife, Bard-Parker knife (blades 11–15)

Castroviejo needle holder, Barraquer-Troutman needle holder and Cohan needle holder

Trephines: Castroviejo set with Weck disposable blades, corneal graft punch (Polack) or corneal block (Kaufman)

Sutures: Dacron 5'0', ¾ circle (for Flieringa rings), 8'0' silk, 9'0' silk (for avascular corneal edema), 10'0' nylon (for most grafts)

I prefer the ethicon GS-10 needles (175° curvature, 7.14 mm long)

Glass syringe, 2-cc, and 30 G cannula, balanced saline irrigator.

PATIENT PREPARATION

The night before surgery, the eyelashes are trimmed and antibiotic drops are applied to the eye. Pilocarpine (1%) drops are applied to the eye before surgery if the eye is phakic. In aphakic eyes, no drops are used; if lens extraction is planned, the pupil is moderately dilated with Neo-synephrine (10%) at the time of surgery if retrobulbar injection has not produced adequate pupil dilation. Almost all cases are done under local anesthesia. The patient receives premedication (Phenergan-Demerol) and oral glycerol (1 gm/kg). In cases when this agent is not indicated, or if the patient cannot drink the glycerol, we start an intravenous infusion of 20% Mannitol 20 min before the actual surgery. In very apprehensive patients, Valium (10 mg) is administered intramuscularly if necessary. An intravenous infusion of normal saline with 5% glucose is kept in place during the surgical procedure.

OPERATIVE TECHNIQUE

The patient receives a Van Lint akinesia and retrobulbar anesthesia, both with 2% xylocaine with adrenaline; in cases of reoperation, 10,000 U of hyaluronidase is mixed with the retrobulbar anesthetic. After inserting a Barraquer wire speculum, a single ring (for phakic cases) is sutured 5 mm from the limbus. Six 5'0' dacron sutures are used to fix the ring to the episclera. Four sutures are left long so they can be secured to the drapes to immobilize the eye in the desired position. In most cases, the speculum can be removed while the lids are retained by the sutures (Fig. 11-3**A**). The host epithelium is not usually removed unless it is very edematous or a fibrovascular membrane covers the cornea. With the ring forceps, the globe is held in position, parallel to the plane of the microscope. A superficial trephination of the cornea is made with a Weck disposable trephine, as shown in Figure 11-3**A**. One or two small drops of methylene blue are placed on the edge of the trephine to help identify the marking on the corneal surface. The use of the disposable blade is of great advantage in centering the trephine over the cornea, a slight tilting of the trephine blade will help to determine the depth of the cut on the cornea. This corneal trephination can easily be localized since it is blue-stained, and deepened if, after removing the trephine, it is found to be too superficial. Ideally, it should be no deeper than one-half the corneal thickness. Following trephination, the corneal cut is deepened with a razor-blade knife with a slight bevel towards the center of the cornea (about 10°) (Fig. 11-3**B**). Once the cut appears to be close to Descemet's membrane all around the cornea, the anterior chamber is penetrated, usually between 9 and 10 o'clock, letting aqueous humor slowly escape through the knife perforation. The cut in Descemet's membrane, however, must be continued for about 5 mm to allow the introduction of a corneal scissors. (Fig. 11-3**C**) With the miniature corneal scissors, the corneal cut is completed, leaving a minimal bevel at the edge of Descemet's membrane. Once the excision of the corneal button is completed, one must check to see if Descemet's membrane has been completely excised or if there are tags or irregular edges in the host border. Should these be present, they are grasped with a jeweler's forceps and sectioned with the Vannas scissors or with the single-curve Castroviejo scissors. One or two iridectomies are performed with the Vannas scissors in grafts over 7.5 mm. In uncomplicated cases where the graft is not larger than 7.5 mm, iridectomy does not seem to be essential;[13,14] therefore, if the displacement of the lens and iris forward makes this iridectomy or iridotomy inconvenient, it should not be attempted. In complicated cases where one expects to perform a graft larger than 8 mm, we prefer to do an ab externo iridectomy at 12 o'clock immediately after outlining the corneal trephination. The anterior chamber is reformed with saline

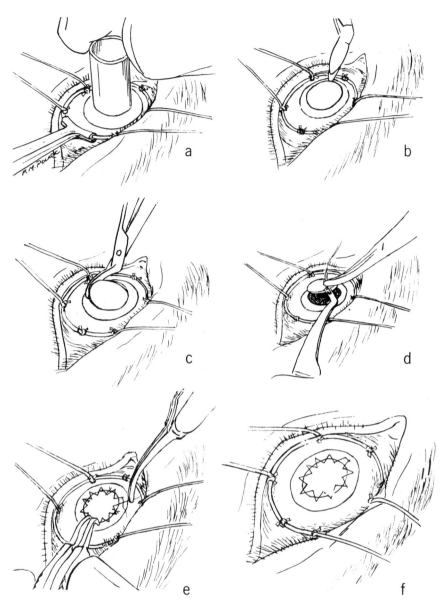

Figure 11-3. Technique for penetrating keratoplasty. **A**. A single Flieringa ring has been sutured to the globe, and it is being held parallel to the microscope with a Llobera-Troutman forceps. A superficial corneal cut is made with an open trephine blade. Staining the edge of the blade with methylene blue facilitates repositioning the trephine and further steps. **B**. With a razor-blade knife, the cut is deepened to almost full-thickness, keeping a slight inward bevel. The anterior chamber is slowly opened to allow the entrance of a corneal scissors. **C**. Excision of the corneal button is completed with scissors that should keep a slight inward inclination. **D**. The first corneal graft suture is placed with a double forceps. The graft should not rest on the iris tissue while the first suture is being placed. **E**. Four cardinal interrupted sutures secure the graft temporarily in place. Monofilament nylon (10′0′) is placed in a continuous fashion. Suture loops are being adjusted before it is tightened near the limbus. **F**. Completed running suture after the four cardinal sutures have been removed.

after the iridectomy, and the wound is closed. Then, the deepening of the corneal cut is made with the blade as described.

Corneas stored in M-K media are placed over the cutting blocks at the time the host cornea is excised, a drop of the media is placed over the cornea, and the tissue is covered with a metallic cup to avoid dehydration or contamination.

In phakic cases, the donor tissue is obtained with a trephine of the same size. Grafts up to the size of 8 mm are cut from the endothelial side over a paraffin or teflon block or with a corneal graft punch (Fig. 11-4 **A** and **B**). The corneal button usually remains over the block, where it is grasped from its edge with the double-pronged forceps on a quadrant away from the operator (Fig. 11-4**C**) in such a way that when the forceps is turned over with the graft to show the epithelial side, it is in the correct position to introduce a silk suture between the two prongs, at the same time avoiding touching the endothelium with any object (Fig. 11-4**D**). Once the needle is partially passed through the graft, it is carried over the host cornea where the first suture is completed (Fig. 11-3**D**). I prefer to place four 8'0' or 9'0' silk sutures in each quadrant before using an interrupted nylon suture. In order to facilitate the handling of the 10'0' nylon material, it is convenient to insert one of the two needles into a small piece of a cellulose sponge so this needle can be easily localized. The first bite of the 10'0' nylon material is placed parallel to the limbus, midway between the corneal section and the limbal area. The purpose of this nonradial bite is to facilitate the beginning of a new graft to host suture in the event that the first suture breaks. Completion of the running nylon suture is done at the limbal suture after tightening the loops (Fig. 11-3 **E** and **F**).

OBTAINING THE GRAFT FOR PENETRATING KERATOPLASTY

The corneal graft can be obtained by trephining the cornea from the epithelial side (Fig. 11-5) or from the endothelial side in the excised cornea as described above.

Possibly, the endothelial cut has more advantages than the epithelial cut, since it minimizes the trauma to the endothelium.[11] Also, it is the only way to cut isolated corneas preserved in tissue culture solutions or cryopreserved corneas. For many years, some European ophthalmologists[6-8] have cut corneal grafts from their endothelial side in order to obtain better, more regular cuts. These surgeons used a paraffin or cork block with a small excavation to set the cornea endothelial side up; the soft block allowed the placement of one or two sutures through the graft edge after its trephination. At the University of Florida, Kaufman et al.[9] used a paraffin block to cut cryopreserved corneas for several years. These blocks were made with laboratory paraffin (69°C) poured in an ice cube tray. Before the blocks hardened, an indentation was made on its surface with a steel ball of a radius of about 8 mm. The blocks were sterilized by immersion in an antiseptic solution. Because paraffin fragments had been found in the anterior chamber of some grafted eyes, we tried other materials, such as

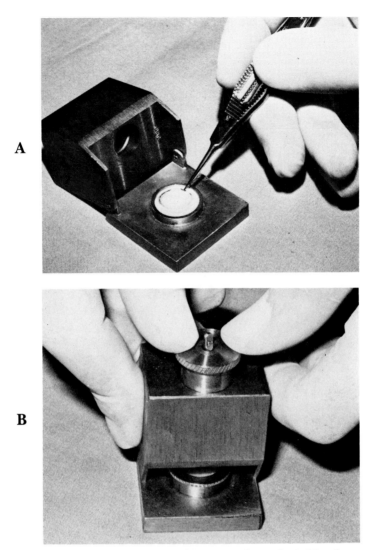

Figure 11-4. Cutting the corneal graft with a corneal punch. **A.** The donor cornea with a scleral ring is positioned in the base of the punch. **B.** The corneal punch being used. **C.** The corneal graft usually remains in the teflon plate. A right-handed operator lifts the

silicone rubber, methyl methacrylate, and teflon (Fig. 11-6 **A** and **C**). The latter gave better results, even though it was hard on the edge of the trephine, but with the advent of disposable trephine blades, this problem was solved. In 1972, we designed a corneal punch[10] (Figs. 11-4 **A** and **B**) to cut these corneas, because the cut with the block often produced oblique graft edges if care was not taken to keep the trephine perpendicular to the cornea. We also found that full trephination of grafts from the epithelial side had to be done against the iris, or if partially cut with the trephine, the excision had to be completed with scissors. In the first event, the graft often rubbed against the iris, losing some cells, and it

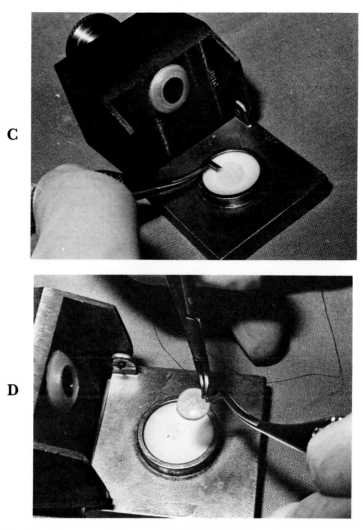

graft with a double-pronged forceps held in his left hand as shown. The tips of the forceps should not touch the graft endothelium. **D**. The surgeon turns over the forceps and the graft in order to insert the first suture through the slit in the forceps. This procedure is usually done over the recipient eye as shown in Figure 11-3**D**.

had to be rinsed with a balanced salt solution to remove iris pigment. If the cut was completed with scissors, the cut was not as regular as the cut from the endothelial side, and a large number of cells were lost at the edge because of scissors trauma.

The corneal punch works well for grafts up to 8.5 mm. Larger grafts require a different base plate (7.5 mm or less), otherwise the graft tends to slide to the center of the 8-mm plate and the cut is not perfectly round. A similar problem may occur with cutting blocks. It is important to keep in mind that with an endothelial cut, it is difficult or impossible to see the extent of the arcus senilis. In

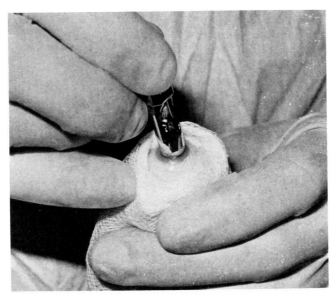

Figure 11-5. A corneal graft being obtained by trephination from the epithelial side. If the cut is made through-and-through, it is necessary to rinse the iris pigment from the graft endothelium. If the trephination is partial, it must be completed with scissors.

an anterior cut, the graft can be decentered, and the arcus avoided. Therefore, for grafts larger than 8 mm, I prefer to cut from the epithelial side, even though a number of endothelial cells will be lost from the borders.

The extreme fragility of endothelial cells can be appreciated in a situation where an endothelial-cut graft was placed over the iris of a keratoconus patient with a fluid layer in between. Because a large arcus was present on the graft, I cut another graft from the mate eye, through the epithelial side and replaced the first graft, which remained over the eye for about 4 min. The first graft was fixed in glutaraldehyde and studied by scanning electron microscope. It showed large areas of endothelial cell loss (Fig. 11-7 **A** and **B**), which corresponded to areas of contact with the iris or to the trauma of depositing the graft over the eye and removing it. In previous experiments, we found no endothelial cell damage in the graft when whole corneas are excised for posterior corneal trephination.[11]

Penetrating keratoplasty gives excellent results in properly selected cases. We like to stress a most careful handling of the graft, good surgical technique, and avoidance of trauma to the recipient eye. Fine's[12] technique of host corneal trephination, as I described in this chapter, is the safest method to open the eye for penetrating keratoplasty.

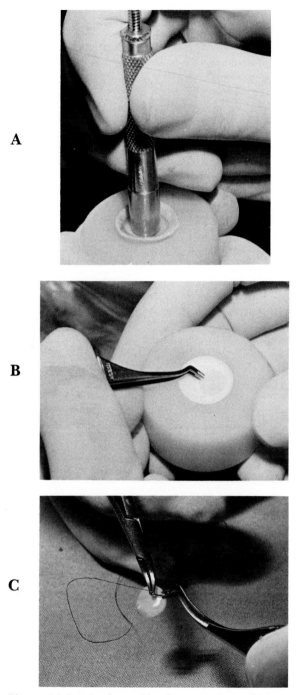

Figure 11-6. Graft trephination on a corneal block. **A**. A trephine with a disposable blade is placed firmly against the cornea, which rests on a teflon block. The trephine must be perpendicular to the cornea. **B**. The graft is lifted from the block with a double forceps, held by the left hand of the surgeon. **C**. The graft is turned over, and the first suture is inserted.

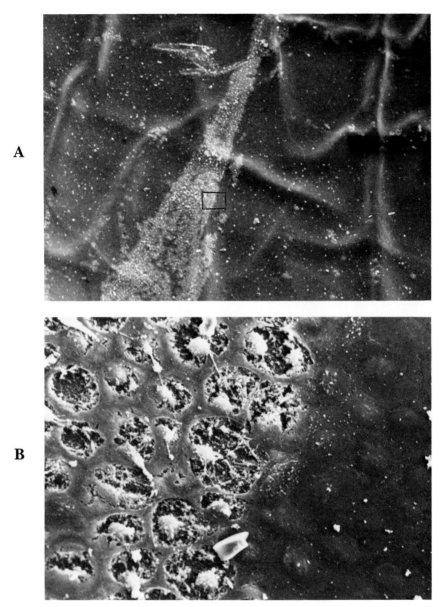

Figure 11-7. **A.** Scanning electron microphotograph of a donor cornea with a localized area of endothelial damage. The square indicates the area magnified in **B** (SEM, ×50). **B.** Magnified area, indicated in **A**, showing areas of endothelial cell destruction. These lesions are not seen in donor corneas excised with proper technique. The defect can be reproduced by endothelial contact with the iris or the edge of the host cornea (SEM, ×1000).

REFERENCES

1. Irvine AR, Kaufman HE: Intraocular pressure following keratoplasty. Am J Ophthalmol 68:835, 1969
2. Gasset AR, Kaufman HE: Hydrophilic lens therapy of severe keratoconjunctivitis sicca and conjunctival scarring. Am J Ophthalmol 71:1185, 1971
3. Polack FM: Current concepts in the management of corneal graft complications, *In* Zimmerman TJ, Kaufman HE (eds): Current Concepts in Ophthalmology, vol V. St. Louis, C.V. Mosby, 1976
4. Polack FM: Lamellar keratoplasty—Malbran's peeling-off technique. Arch Ophthalmol 86:293, 1971
5. Harms H, Mackensen G: Ocular Surgery Under the Microscope. Chicago, Yearbook Medical, 1967
6. Vannas M: Remarks on the technique of corneal transplantation, *In* Paton RT (ed): Keratoplasty, New York, McGraw Hill, 1955, pp 151. Am J Ophthalmol 33:70, 1950
7. Masler M: Cited by: Kadlecova V. The profile of the circular corneal transplant. (abstr.) Excerpta Medica 4:282, 1950
8. Stallard HB: Eye Surgery. Baltimore, Williams & Wilkins, 1958, p 415
9. Capella JA, Kaufman HE, Robbins JE: Preservation of viable corneal tissue. Cryobiology 2:116, 1965
10. Polack FM, Capella JA: A corneal punch. Am J Ophthalmol 67:966, 1969
11. Brightbill FS, Polack FM, Slappey T: A comparison of two methods of cutting donor corneal buttons. Am J Ophthalmol 74:500, 1973
12. Fine M: Technique of penetrating keratoplasty, *In*: Dabezies OH, Gitter KA, Samson CLM (eds): Symposium of the Cornea, New Orleans Academy of Ophthalmology. St. Louis, C.V. Mosby, 1972, p 132
13. Galvao PG: Transplante de cornea, thesis. Facultade de medicina da Univ. Fed. Minas Gerais. Belo Horizonte, Brazil, 1976
14. Rice NS: The prognosis for penetrating keratoplasty. Trans Ophthalmol Soc 94:94, 1974

Chapter 12

Keratoplasty in Aphakia; Keratoplasty and Lens Extraction

Prior to 1950, results of penetrating keratoplasty in aphakic eyes were discouraging.[1-5] At that time, corneal surgeons were still using small grafts (3–5 mm), secured to the host by appositional sutures or a conjunctival flap. Most of these grafts were bound to fail because of poor apposition and vitreous prolapse. Early in the 1950s, however, good results were reported by Stocker[6] in eyes with corneal edema due to Fuchs' dystrophy. Following this report, others reported successful grafts in aphakia.[7-13] Among the several factors that improved the prognosis in these eyes were, the use of larger grafts, the development of finer needles and instrumentation, "edge-to-edge" suturing, recognition and treatment of preoperative glaucoma, and aspiration-excision of vitreous from the wound area. Thus, Fine,[14] using a new surgical technique, was able to report good results in 70%–90% of unfavorable and favorable cases,[15,16] a figure similar to that obtained today by other surgeons.[17,18]

PREOPERATIVE CONSIDERATIONS

The most common condition requiring keratoplasty in aphakic eyes is corneal edema. A minor number of cases are due to corneal scarring or ulcerations. It is accepted that corneal edema is due to endothelial dystrophy (Fuchs') or decompensation following cataract extraction or intraocular inflammation. In most instances, endothelial disease after cataract extraction is more common than Fuchs' dystrophy;[15] however, in advanced cases of severe edema with vascularization and scarring, the diagnosis can be made only after histologic study of the excised tissue.

Functional rehabilitation of the eye can be obtained only by a penetrating keratoplasty. Lamellar grafts have no place in the therapy of this disease, except for symptomatic treatment for an undetermined period of time. Results of keratoplasty depend on the preoperative status of the eye. An arbitrary classification in three groups is convenient for final prognosis.

Group I: Favorable cases. Cases presenting several of the following: edema, mostly in the central portion; round pupil; vitreous face intact; normal intraocular pressure and deep anterior chamber; peripheral corneal thickness between 0.7 and 0.8 mm (measured 2 mm inside the limbus). (Prognosis Index 71, see chapter 13.)

Group II: Moderately favorable cases. These cases are characterized by corneal edema extending to the limbus with peripheral thickness estimated between 0.8 and 0.9 mm; deformed pupil with vitreous adhesions to the cornea; superficial stromal vessels; moderate elevation of intraocular pressure controllable with medication. (Prognosis Index 64, see chapter 13.)

Group III: Unfavorable cases. Unfavorable prognosis is based on advanced corneal edema with deep vessels; thickness at periphery estimated at 1 mm or more; vitreous adhesions to cornea; severe glaucoma; history of uveitis; reoperations with evidence of retrocorneal membrane. (Prognosis Index 49, see chapter 13.)

The presence of a cataract in groups I and II does not seem to modify its prognosis when a combined keratoplasty and cataract extraction is done. It appears, however, that the complications related to vitrectomy (most commonly, macular edema) and vitreous contact to the graft can be eliminated by extracapsular lens extraction.

PREPARATION OF HOST EYE PRIOR TO KERATOPLASTY

Patients in categories II and III may require preoperative therapy for glaucoma control and reduction of corneal edema. Intraocular pressure determinations are made with the MacKay-Marg tonometer or an air tonometer.[21] Cryotherapy of the ciliary body 2 or 3 wk before keratoplasty is perhaps the most useful way of decreasing the intraocular pressure when medical therapy fails; however, in several cases, we have done filtering operations (subscleral sclerectomy) previous to corneal grafting. In cases of severe edema and large bullae, diathermy cauterization of Bowman's membrane[19,20] is done 2–3 wk prior to keratoplasty. This procedure decreases corneal edema and facilitates the alignment of the graft.

Bacterial cultures are taken 1 or 2 wk preoperatively. Only those eyes harboring pathogenic bacteria are treated.

The patient receives glycerol orally (1 g/kg) 1½–2 hr preoperatively and is premedicated for local anesthesia. The degree of hypotony is checked again in the operating room, and if necessary, intravenous mannitol 20% (1 g/kg) is administered. The pupil is not dilated before surgery.

OPERATIVE TECHNIQUE

A Barraquer lid speculum or lid sutures are used. A double Flieringa ring is sutured to the episclera with 5'0' dacron or silk sutures as shown in Figure 12-1**A**. It is effective to also suture the large ring to add extra support to the scleral wall. The speculum can be removed.

A graft of 7.5 mm is preferred, since it should contain enough healthy endothelium to restore the corneal function and still would permit the use of a larger graft if a reoperation is required. The loose and edematous epithelium of the recipient eye is gently removed with a scalpel. A superficial cut (0.3 mm) is

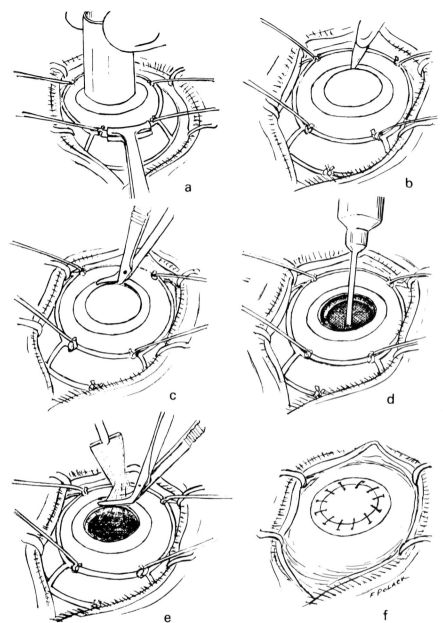

a

b

c

d

e

f

Figure 12-1. **A.** A double Flieringa ring has been sutured to the episcleral tissue of the eye. Long sutures are secured to the drapes with clamps. A partial trephination (⅓) of the cornea is performed with trephine blade (stained with methylene blue) under direct microscopic observation. **B.** The area of trephination is deepened (⅔) with a razor-blade knife. The chamber is entered with the knife. **C.** The corneal button is excised with scissors making a slight inward bevel. **D.** Fluid vitreous is being aspirated with a 22-G needle. **E.** Formed vitreous and vitreous over the iris is excised with scissors while being lifted with cellulose sponges. The wound edges must be free of vitreous. **F.** The graft is sutured in place with deep, interrupted 9′0′ silk sutures (GS-10) in cases of severe corneal edema; otherwise, continuous monofilament 10′0′ nylon is used.

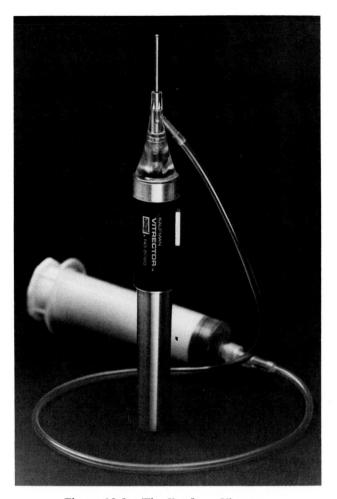

Figure 12-2. The Kaufman Vitrector

made in the cornea with a trephine blade that has been stained with 1%
methylene blue. Then, the superficial cut is deepened with a razor-blade knife,
making a slight inward bevel (Fig. 12-1**B**). The chamber is entered with the
blade, and the cut is slowly enlarged to 2 or 3 mm, so a corneal scissors can be
inserted. The button is completely excised (Fig. 12-1**C**). If necessary, one or
more iridotomies are done with sharp scissors. If vitreous is adherent to the
corneal button, it is sectioned with curved scissors. After the button is removed,
fluid vitreous is aspirated through the pupil with a 22-G needle (Fig. 12-1**D**) so
the iris diaphragm recedes to the vitreous cavity (usually 0.5 cc). Formed vitreous
must be removed from the anterior chamber and iris surface with the aid of
cellulose sponges and scissors (Fig. 12-1**E**), and any strands present at the wound
edge must be removed with a vitrectomy instrument, such as the Kaufman
Vitrector (Fig. 12-2), or with the Girard-Sparta Phaco-Fragmentation Unit (Fig.
12-3). The donor material may be fresh or cryopreserved tissue that is cut 0.5

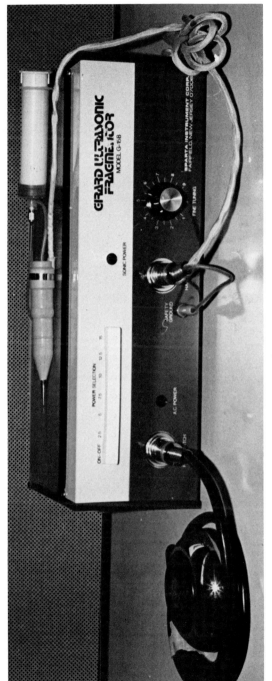

Figure 12-3. The Girard-Sparta Phaco-Fragmentation Unit.

153

mm larger than the host from the endothelial side on a teflon block. The graft is then held with a fine double forceps to avoid undue trauma to the graft endothelium at the time of inserting the first suture and, moreover, to avoid dipping the graft into the eye and contaminating it with vitreous. If fresh tissue is used and cut from the epithelial side, the insertion of two sutures at opposite ends at the time of cutting facilitates suturing. As previously mentioned, we prefer the endothelial side cut because it is less traumatic than scissors, and the tissue obtains a more perpendicular cut, which favors a better closure of the posterior wound. For this reason, I use this method for fresh tissue.

The suture material should stimulate scarring to some degree; therefore, silk is preferred for edematous corneas. Virgin 8'0' and 9'0' silk (GS-10) are the two most frequently used materials, with the sutures placed very deep (Fig. 12-1F). However, in cases with moderate edema or stromal vascularization, we use 10'0' continuous nylon suture (GS-14). Artificial aqueous humor, often with a small air bubble, is injected into the anterior chamber with a 30-G needle at the conclusion of the operation. Utilizing the microscope, the wound is tested for leaks by gently pressing around the graft with a cellulose sponge. The ring is removed, subconjunctival Gentamicin (20 mg) and Solu-Medrol (10 mg) are injected, as well as atropine drops.

KERATOPLASTY AND LENS EXTRACTION

A decision for lens extraction is usually done before surgery; however, sometimes the advanced degree of corneal edema requires a decision in the operating room. Once the corneal button is removed, one can obtain an idea of lens changes by using the coaxial light of the microscope after filling the anterior chamber with balanced saline solution. In practice, we usually remove the lens of patients over 60 yr of age. In this study, all extractions were intracapsular. The pupil was not dilated before surgery, and lens extraction was done with a cryoextractor applied to the central portion of the lens. In several cases, chymotrypsin was used, but generally, the mechanical rupture of the zonula was satisfactory.[30] Acetylocholine (Miochol) was used after lens extraction. One or two peripheral iridectomies were done with Vannas scissors before the graft was sutured in place. If vitrectomy was not required, no atropine was used at the end of the procedure. Routinely, we use subconjunctival steroids and Gentamicin.

Table 12-1 indicates that from a group of 85 consecutive cases operated on at the University of Florida, 72% from the "favorable" group showed improvement. In group II, (moderately favorable), 43% were improved. Patients in group III (unfavorable) were separated into a group with light-perception vision and another with finger counting vision preoperatively. Only 42% of the cases in group III with finger counting vision were improved. In this group, glaucoma was present in most of the eyes prior to surgery; and even when the glaucoma was controlled, the final results were not satisfactory. There were 11 patients in Group III with light-perception vision (Table 12-2), and all except two had corneal edema. Seventy percent of all patients had clear grafts (Fig. 12-4), and vision was improved in 54% of the cases. From 6 months to 1 yr postoperatively, advanced glaucoma, vitreous hemorrhage, and late expulsive hemorrhage were

Table 12-1
Aphakic Grafts

Group	I	II	IIIA	IIIB
Average preoperative vision	20/100	Hand motion	Finger counting	Light perception
Number of cases	18	37	19	11
Average postoperative vision	20/60	20/40	20/40	20/100
Improved	(13) 72%	(16) 43%	(8) 42%	(6) 54%
Number with previous glaucoma	6	6	12	4

causes of failure (1 case). Cryopreserved tissue was used in seven patients, and fresh tissue in four cases. Table 12-3 shows that the most frequent complications in the early postoperative period are synechiae, glaucoma, vitreous contact to the graft, macular edema, and intraocular hemorrhage. Late complications (over 6 mo) included glaucoma, synechiae, macular edema, retrocorneal membrane formation, graft rejection, and retinal detachment.

Table 12-2
Aphakic Grafts, Group III (Preoperative Vision: Light Perception)

Age	Glaucoma Preop	Postop	Tissue	Size	Combined	Clear	VA (6 mo)	Improved
71	+	+	Cryo	9.0	+	+	20/200	+
68	−		Cryo	8.0	−	+	20/200	+
72	−		Cryo	7.5	−	−	HM	−
49*	−	+	Cryo	9.0	−	+	LP (Gl)	−
69	+	+	Cryo	7.5	−	+	LP (Gl)	−
31*	−		Cryo	7.5	+	+	HM (Mac)	+
67	−		Cryo	8.0	+	−	HM	+
72	+	+	Fresh	7.5	−	+	FC	+
65	−		Fresh	7.5	−	−	Exp Hem	−
72	−		Fresh	8.0	−	+	20/100	+
42	+	+	Fresh	7.5	+	+	LP (Vit Hem)	−
	4				4	8		6

70% of the grafts were clear.
54% had improved vision.
*Had combined cataract extraction and graft. VA, visual acuity; LP, light perception; FC, finger counting; Exp Hem, expulsive hemorrhage; Vit Hem, vitreous hemorrhage; HM, hand motion; Gl, glaucoma; Mac, macular degeneration.

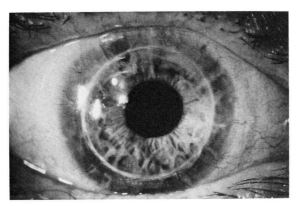

Figure 12-4. A clear 8-mm penetrating keratoplasty in an aphakic eye 6 mo after surgery.

Penetrating keratoplasty in aphakia is indicated in cases of pain and/or poor vision bilaterally. Monocular edema is usually treated conservatively. Our results show that in an unfavorable group of cases with advanced corneal disease, two of which had a cataract removed at the time of grafting and several with glaucoma, clear grafts were obtained in 70% of the cases, with visual improvement in 6 of 11 patients. This figure is compatible with results reported by Fine[14,15] of 87% or better results in favorable cases and results of 60% and 50%, respectively, in unfavorable cases with severe corneal edema after cataract extraction and preexisting glaucoma. Buxton[22] reports 80% clear grafts after cataract extraction and only 56% in combined keratoplasty and cataract extraction. In this small number of cases (Table 12-2), two grafts remained clear after cataract extraction was done simultaneously with keratoplasty.

It is our impression that this combined procedure does not decrease the chance of a clear graft. Preoperative hypotony with vitreous aspiration is recognized as being of prime importance[23,24] as well as the use of fresh and healthy donor tissue and the control of postoperative inflammation to protect the endothelium.[25] It is accepted that previous glaucoma, usually of a secondary type, decreases the percentage of clear grafts,[15] an observation that we have been able to confirm in this series. (Table 12-1). It is now accepted that transplanted

Table 12-3
Complications

Early (0–6 mo)	Late (>6 mo)
Synechiae	Glaucoma
Glaucoma	Macular edema
Vitreous contact	Synechiae
Macular edema	Retrocorneal membrane (vitreous contact)
Vitreous hemorrhage	Graft rejection
Expulsive hemorrhage	Retinal detachment

endothelial cells can survive for long periods of time, if not indefinitely, in the new host.[26]

Transplantation of donor tissue with poor endothelial viability, with much surgical trauma (particularly at the edges), accounts for postoperative edema of the graft and early failure. A properly handled graft should survive; however, Stocker[27] believed that grafts in aphakic eyes had a limited survival time, even if done without surgical complication.

After reviewing regrafted specimens, it appears that early as well as later graft edema is caused by vitreous contact to the endothelium with gradual destruction of these cells and eventual replacement by connective tissue (see chapter 15). Clinically, this shows initially as a loss of the crystalline transparency of the graft and later by haziness and edema (Fig. 12-5). Histologically, one finds a fine membrane replacing areas devoid of endothelial cells[28] or retrocorneal membranes similar to that described by Snip and Kenyon.[29]

Technically, grafts in aphakia are not more complicated than keratoplasties in phakic eyes; however, special consideration must be given to the degree of corneal edema, so deep sutures must be applied to properly align the posterior layers of the graft with the host endothelium. Aspiration or removal of vitreous strands from the trephination area is extremely important, and the use of a surgical microscope facilitates these two steps. The use of silk sutures assures faster healing, so after 4 mo, sutures can be removed. To obviate the slower healing of wounds with 10'0' nylon, Kaufman[30] uses a second continuous suture of 15-μ nylon, which is left in place permanently after the thicker nylon is removed (Fig. 12-6).

The other factors that have improved the results in this type of surgery are the recognition of preoperative glaucoma in eyes with edematous corneas and also postoperative glaucoma.[16,21] The feasibility of measuring this pressure in recently operated eyes, the use of hyperosmotic agents, and carbonic anhydrase inhibitors has unquestionably improved the results of transplantation. The deleterious effect of increased intraocular pressure on corneal endothelium has been pointed out by Svedberg.[31] Recently, R. Olson (personal communication,

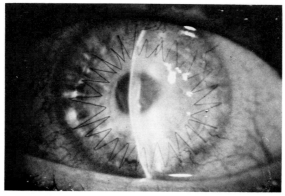

Figure 12-5. A 7-mo-old graft with progressive edema due to diffuse vitreous contact.

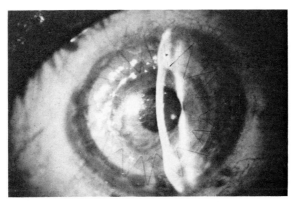

Figure 12-6. Two sets of continuous nylon sutures (10'0' and 15-μ).

1977) has found that postoperative glaucoma can be eliminated by using grafts larger (0.5 to 1 mm) than the host's window.

From this study, therefore, it appears that results of penetrating kerato-plasty in aphakic eyes, particularly in bullous keratopathy, are comparable to those obtained in phakic eyes.[32] On the basis of the degree of corneal disease, pathologic changes in the anterior segment, and glaucoma, cases can be given various prognoses. In this series of 85 consecutive patients with various clinical prognoses, there were 70% clear grafts between 6 mo and 1 yr postoperatively.

KERATOPLASTY WITH EXTRACAPSULAR LENS EXTRACTION

The development of macular edema and other vitreo–retinal problems as-sociated with anterior vitrectomies has not been adequately evaluated in the series described above. These complications, as well as graft edema (possibly due to vitreous contact) were rather frequent and required a modification in our technique. Ten grafts were done during the period of 1976–1977 in combination with an extracapsular cataract extraction. In these cases, the pupil was dilated before surgery, the corneal button excised, and a large anterior capsulotomy done in a circular manner with a razor-blade knife and scissors. The nucleus is extracted with a cystotome or expressed with a spatula and a lens loop. Cortical material is removed with a bulb irrigator. Peripheral cortical fibers are best removed with an olive-tipped needle attached to a 2-cc syringe filled with bal-anced saline (Fig. 12-7). While an assistant fills the anterior chamber with bal-anced salt solution, a gentle aspiration–inspiration ("push–pull") technique will detach and peel away material attached to the lens capsule. The central portion of the capsule can be scraped with a capsule spatula (Sparta-Girard). Acetyl-choline (Miochol) is then instilled, and one or two peripheral iridectomies are done before graft suturing. This technique has produced results superior to those of previous techniques in this group of patients because increased in-traocular pressure has been minimal or absent and macular edema has not been observed.

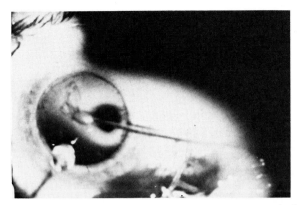

Figure 12-7. Peripheral cortical fibers being removed with an olive-tipped needle attached to a 2-cc syringe filled with balanced saline solution.

REFERENCES

1. Owens WC: Symposium on corneal transplantation. Am J Ophthalmol 31:1394, 1948
2. Franceschetti A: Corneal grafting. Trans Ophthalmol Soc UK 69:17, 1949
3. Castroviejo R: Indications and contraindications for keratoplasty and keratectomies. Am J Ophthalmol 29:1081, 1946
4. Roberts JE: Statistics on results of keratoplasty. Am J Ophthalmol 33:21, 1950
5. Paufique L, Sourdille GP, Offret G: Les Greffes de la Corneé. Paris, Masson et Cie, 1948
6. Stocker FW: Successful corneal grafts in the care of endothelial and epithelial corneal dystrophy. Am J Ophthalmol 35:349, 1952
7. Thomas JWT: Technique and results in keratoplasty. Trans Ophthalmol Soc UK 75:473, 1955
8. Casey TA: Penetrating keratoplasty in aphakia. Trans Ophthalmol Soc UK 81:705, 1961
9. Doctor DW, Traynor EM: Penetrating keratoplasty in Fuchs' endothelial dystrophy. Am J Ophthalmol 54:812, 1962
10 Hughes, WF: The treatment of corneal dystrophies by keratoplasty. Am J Ophthalmol 50:1100, 1960
11. Fine M: Therapeutic keratoplasty, Symposium: Corneal surgery. Trans Am Acad Ophthalmol Otolaryngol 64:786, 1960
12. Paton RT: Keratoplasty. New York, Blackinston, 1955
13. Ganther G: Late results of 100 successful keratoplasties. Dtsch Ophthalmol Ges 64:159, 1961
14. Fine M: Penetrating keratoplasty in aphakia. Arch Ophthalmol 72:50, 1964
15. Fine M: Keratoplasty in aphakia, *In* King J, McTigue J (eds): The Corneal World Congress. Washington, Butterworths, 1965, pp 538–552
16. Fine M: Corneal grafts and aphakia, *In* Rycoff PR (ed): Corneo-Plastic Surgery, Proceedings of the Second International Congress. London, Pergamon, 1969, p 289
17. Kaufman HE, Capella J, Polack FM: Keratoplasty with refrigerated and cryopreserved donor tissue, *In* Capella J, Edelhausertt, and Van Horne D (eds): *Corneal Preservation.* Springfield, Ill., Charles C Thomas, 1971, p 191

18. Sanders N: Penetrating corneal transplants for aphakic bullous keratopathy. South Med J 61:869, 1968
19. Salleras A: Bullous keratopathy, *In* King J, McTigue J (eds): The Cornea World Congress. Washington, Butterworths, 1965, p 292
20. DeVoe AG: Electrocautery of Bowman's membrane. Arch Ophthalmol 76:768, 1966
21. Irvine AR, Kaufman HE: Intraocular pressure following penetrating keratoplasty. Am J Ophthalmol 68:835, 1969
22. Buxton JN: Non-simultaneous and simultaneous corneal graft and cataract extraction, *In* Polack FM (ed): Corneal and External Diseases of the Eye. Springfield, Ill, Charles C Thomas, 1970, p 243
23. Castroviejo R: Penetrating grafting—Regrafting and unusual cases, *In* King J, McTigue J (eds): The Cornea World Congress. Washington, Butterworths, 1965, pp 553–563
24. Barraquer J: Present status of corneal transplant surgery. Highl Ophthalmol 5:320, 1962
25. Dohlman CH, Boruchoff AS: Penetrating keratoplasty, *In* Dohlman CH (ed): Corneal Edema, Boston, Little, Brown, 1968, p 655
26. Polack FM, Smelser GK: Long-term survival of isotopically labelled stromal and endothelial cells in corneal homografts. Am J Ophthalmol 57:67, 1964
27. Stocker FW, Irish A: Ultimate fate of successful corneal grafts done for endothelial dystrophy (Fuchs'). Trans Ophthalmol Soc 67:196, 1969
28. Polack FM: Discussion, in "Retrocorneal membrane," (Contreras F), *In* Polack FM (ed): Corneal and External Diseases of the Eye. Springfield, Ill, Charles C Thomas, 1970, p 142
29. Snip RC, Kenyon KR, Green WR: Retrocorneal fibrous membrane in the vitreous touch syndrome. Am J Ophthalmol 79:233, 1975
30. Kaufman HE: Combined keratoplasty and cataract extraction. Am J Ophthalmol 77:824, 1974
31. Svedberg B: Effects of artificial intraocular pressure elevation on the outflow facility and the ultrastructure of the chamber angle in the vervet monkey. Acta Ophthalmol 52:829, 1974
32. Polack FM: Penetrating keratoplasty in aphakia. Rev Soc Col Oftalmol 2:200, 1971

Part 3

Influence of Host Response in Clinical Results and Pathology of the Graft

Chapter 13

Influence of Host Corneal Disease in the Prognosis of Keratoplasty

Anatomical alterations of the host cornea may cause healing problems that may eventually be the cause of graft opacification, including the immune reaction. Even though a meticulous surgical technique is available, many surgeons like to assess or evaluate the eye to be grafted and expect or predict a certain degree of graft success. Evaluation of the recipient cases as "very favorable," "favorable," or "unfavorable" for penetrating keratoplasty has been done in the past by Castroviejo.[1,2] This classification is useful, but with the availability of finer sutures and steroids in recent years, cases with poor prognosis have moved to a better category.

Changes in corneal structure will increase graft coaptation problems. Other alterations that may affect graft healing include: (A) hyperplastic epithelium and anterior fibrous membrane (Fig. 13-1); (B) thick or thin stroma; (C) active stromal inflammation; and (D) retrocorneal fibrous membrane and iris synechiae or pigmented membrane (Fig. 13-2). Additional changes that will have an important bearing on the fate of the graft, particularly on the development of graft rejections are deep stromal vascularization and neoformation of lymphatic channels in the stroma. Khodadoust[3] has pointed out the importance of stromal vessels in the development of homograft reactions, an observation shared by Fine and Stein[4] and by us.[5] Recently, it has been considered that these corneas deserve tissue typing if one expects to reduce the incidence of rejection.[6] Localized and avascular lesions or certain groups of corneal dystrophies or degenerations will have more favorable prognosis, one of them being keratoconus, as long as there is moderate variation in thickness from host to graft. Paton[7] has called attention to the importance of host structure in graft prognosis, particularly corneal thickness and vascularization. Keratoconus patients have an exaggerated vascular and inflammatory response, and it is well known that many have multiple allergies and are prone to develop immune reactions. Based on the above mentioned facts, the prognosis of corneal grafts can be divided into several groups, as follows (Table 13-1):

Favorable cases grade I. In addition to keratoconus, other favorable cases are corneal scars due to trauma and scars resulting from bacterial or fungal infections (Fig. 13-3**A–F**) once the inflammatory process has been controlled. I prefer to wait at least 6 mo after the healing of corneal inflammatory lesions before attempting corneal surgery. Herpetic scars, if avascular and inactive for many months, are also favorable for penetrating keratoplasty. Good results are expected in over 90% of these cases.

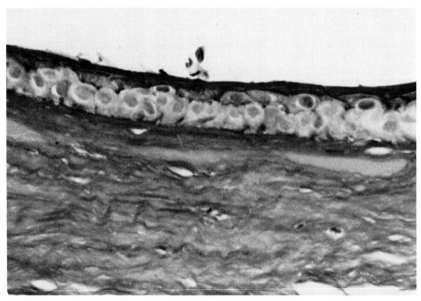

Figure 13-1. Subepithelial fibrous membrane and destruction of Bowman's membrane in a case of chronic keratitis (PAS, ×400).

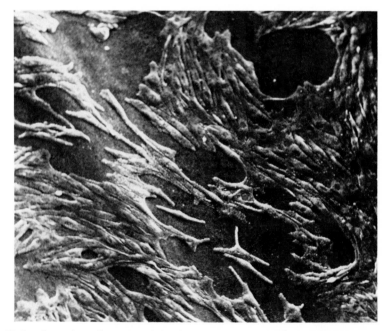

Figure 13-2. Scanning electron microphotograph of a pigmented retrocorneal membrane. This membrane is formed by iris melanocytes spreading over Descemet's membrane (SEM, ×2000).

Table 13-1
Prognosis of Corneal Grafts

Favorable	I.	Avascular corneal scars, keratoconus
	II.	Stromal dystrophies
	III.	Mildly vascularized scars, Fuchs' dystrophy (moderate), inactive herpetic scars
Intermediate	I.	Advanced Fuchs' dystrophy, congenital anomalies with partially absent endothelium without glaucoma
	II.	Moderate anterior segment pathology and glaucoma
	III.	Moderate stromal vascularization and scarring, moderately dry eyes, moderate (superficial or localized) chemical burns
Unfavorable	I.	Very thin or very thick corneas (edema and posterior corneal membrane), active keratitis (viral, bacterial or immunoallergic), uveitis, severe corneal vascularization, anterior segment disease or necrosis that requires total keratoplasty, congenital edema, advanced severe eye dryness
	II.	Severe chemical burns, severe glaucoma and anterior segment synechiae, radiation keratitis, epithelization of anterior chamber and cornea

Favorable cases grade II.   Here we may include many stromal dystrophies without vascularization, such as granular, macular, lattice, and crystalline dystrophies. Even though immediate and long-term results have been excellent in many of these patients, the background metabolic alteration may eventually affect the graft as it has been recently documented.[8] Results here showed approximately 90% clear grafts.

Favorable cases grade III.   Mildly vascularized corneas without active inflammation, inactive herpes, Fuchs' endothelial dystrophy of moderate degree, and failed grafts from the two preceding groups may be classified here. Results varying from 70%–80% clear grafts can be expected.

Moderately favorable cases or intermediate group.   Here we may consider the group of eyes with associated alterations in the anterior segment that may induce the reactivation of previous inflammation, eyes with secondary glaucoma under control, moderately dry eyes, and regraft cases from the previous groups (Fig. 13-4 **A–C**). Late results may yield 40%–60% clear grafts.

Unfavorable cases grade I.   Extremely thin or thick corneas, active corneal inflammation or iritis, severe glaucoma, deep vascularization with firm scar tissue, anterior synechiae, and congenital corneal edema are included here. Thin, fibrotic corneas are particularly prone to cause complications because of their tendency to persistent leakage around sutures and slow healing. (Fig. 13-5 **A–F**)

Unfavorable cases grade II.   This grade encompasses severe corneal vascularization with thinning or soft stromal tissue (chemical burn) usually associated

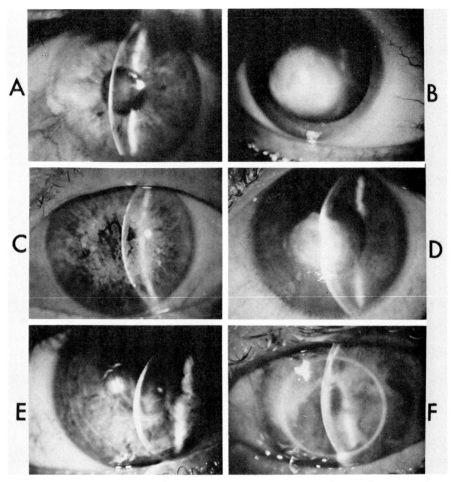

Figure 13-3. Examples of favorable cases for penetrating keratoplasty. **A.** Central corneal scar, secondary to a fungal infection. **B.** Traumatic corneal scar with mild lens changes. **C.** Granular corneal dystrophy. **D.** Herpetic corneal ulceration in remission. **E.** Fuchs' endothelial dystrophy. **F.** Failed graft in a case of herpetic keratitis; because of the lack of deep vascularization the prognosis in this case is relatively good.

with anterior segment pathology (retrocorneal membrane, peripheral anterior synechiae, cataract, etc.), active keratitis with stromal necrosis, radiation keratitis with necrosis, and epithelization of the anterior chamber (Fig. 13-6 **A–D**). The percentage of clear grafts in unfavorable hosts is variable, but rarely will exceed 40–50%.

    Proper evaluation of these cases may help to predict the fate of the graft and prevent complications, such as herpetic reinfection, wound dehiscence, ulcerations, edema, etc. Aronson and Moore's classification of corneal disease[9] offers prognosis based on structural host changes (0 = best, 5 = worst). Sometimes, surgery preparatory to penetrating keratoplasty in the form of keratectomy, superficial Bowman's cautery (Salleras procedure[23]), lamellar grafts, or conjunctivoplasty with limited use of beta therapy may shift a case to a more favorable group.[1]

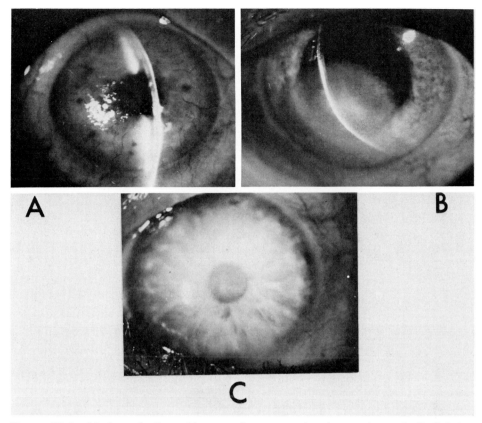

Figure 13-4. Moderately favorable cases for penetrating keratoplasty. **A.** Fuchs' dystrophy in an aphakic eye with moderate degree of deep stromal vascularization. **B.** Corneal scar following Pseudomonas infection; the scar is avascular; however, the cornea is extremely thin in the area of opacification. **C.** Advanced Fuchs' endothelial dystrophy with pronounced stromal thickening.

From all these intermediate or unfavorable host conditions that may influence the fate of the graft, there are some that, in our experience, are more common, such as herpetic keratitis and corneal vascularization. Others are not so frequently seen, but their treatment is more difficult or challenging, as in the case of epithelization of the anterior chamber and chemical burns with subsequent formation of retrocorneal fibrous membranes. Glaucoma is another preoperative condition that may be overlooked in many cases because the pressure is not adequately measured with most clinical instruments.

PROGNOSIS OF PENETRATING KERATOPLASTY—
AN OBJECTIVE EVALUATION

It is evident that even though there are many pathologic conditions in the host eye that will influence the results of keratoplasty, other factors are equally important in obtaining clear grafts, such as the skill of the surgeon or the quality

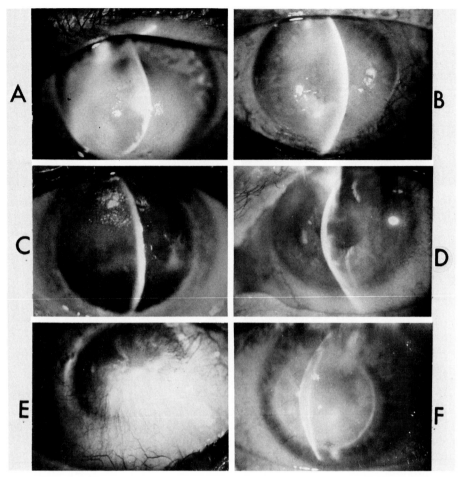

Figure 13-5. **A.** Severe corneal hydrops with corneal thinning to the inferior limbus. **B.** Corneal edema secondary to herpetic uveitis and glaucoma. **C.** Chronic keratitis in a case of Sjögren's disease. **D.** Corneal edema with lens luxation, vitreous adhesion, stromal vascularization, and glaucoma. **E.** Corneal scar and symblepharon following chemical burn. **F.** Failed graft with dense retrocorneal membrane and deep vascularization.

of the donor tissue. It seemed unfair, therefore, to judge potential results from what we routinely classify as a favorable or unfavorable case without rating the severity of important factors (vascularization, glaucoma, etc.). With so many variables, it is obvious that what is a poor prognosis case for one surgeon might be a favorable case for another. In order to solve this evaluation problem, Dr. Donald Willard suggested the development of a system to objectively determine the prognosis for success of a corneal graft. We developed a Prognosis Index (PI), which can be arranged by each individual surgeon (Table 13-2).

Table 13-2 takes into account the principles present in various chapters of this book, such as the skill of the surgeon and his ability to perform atraumatic surgery under the microscope, his knowledge of factors that influence tissue repair, background in corneal pathology, etc. Documentation of the importance

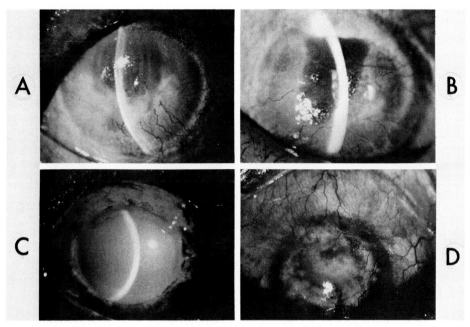

Figure 13-6. A. Corneal edema with stromal vascularization and glaucoma. **B.** Post-traumatic epithelization of the anterior chamber with stromal edema and vascularization. **C.** Total corneal opacification following chemical burn. **D.** Repeated graft failure in a case of chemical injury.

Table 13-2
Graft Prognosis Index: Ten Factors

Factors	Maximum Points
1. Surgeon	10
2. Donor tissue	10
3. No A. C. inflammation	10
4. No host vessels	10
5. No thinning or thickening	10
6. Normal endothelium (peripheral)	10
7. Normal epithelium (to limbus)	10
8. Normal tear film	10
9. Normal intraocular pressure	10
10. No surgical complications	10
Total possible points	100

The prognosis of successful keratoplasty is as follows:

81–100 points	Excellent
71–80 points	Good
51–70 points	Fair
50 points or less	Poor

of first-class donor tissue and the importance of abnormal conditions (in the cornea and the eye itself) are discussed in other chapters. Paton has also elaborated a point system to estimate final prognosis of grafts based on three important ancillary factors: glaucoma, tear film and lid function, and patient compliance.[7]

Table 13-2 lists 10 important factors for determining the prognosis of a successful corneal graft. Grading is done from 0 (worst) to 10 (best). The most important factor is the donor tissue, and points should not be less than 8, as this would correspond to tissue of borderline viability. The definition of ideal donor tissue (10 points) is a cornea below age 50 and less than 10 hr postmortem. Vitreous in the anterior chamber (pre- or intraoperatively) is considered a surgical complication, resulting in a value of no more than 5 points of the possible 10.

Examples

(1) Post-cataract bullous keratopathy.   Corneal edema to limbus, moderate deep vascularization, glaucoma under control, vitreous adherent to cornea. Donor tissue is less than 10 hr post mortem.

1— 7 points	
2—10 points	
3— 6 points	
4— 5 points	
5— 8 points	Total points: 67
6— 2 points	Prognosis: Fair
7— 5 points	
8—10 points	
9— 9 points	
10— 5 points	

(2) Chemical burn, dry eye, uveitis, and glaucoma. The cornea has a thickness of 0.3 mm, and it is vascularized. Peripheral synechiae and cataract are present.

1—10 points	
2—10 points	
3— 2 points	
4— 0 points	
5— 0 points	Total points: 34
6— 0 points	Prognosis: Poor
7— 0 points	
8— 2 points	
9— 5 points	
10— 5 points	

HERPETIC KERATITIS AND
KERATOPLASTY—EXPERIMENTAL STUDIES

Herpetic keratitis and herpetic infections of corneal grafts form a special group of problems in spite of newer antiviral agents. It is important to understand some of the background of the disease in order to be able to manage these cases adequately. In this and the following chapters, we will discuss the various factors that seem to influence the graft survival in herpes-infected hosts.

In an attempt to answer the question of incidence of graft rejection in cases of herpetic keratitis, Wind et al.[10] made reference to a clinical study of Polack and Kaufman,[11] where they reported a low incidence of graft rejection in eyes with previous herpetic keratitis. In a series of experiments in rabbits, they tried to determine the fate of penetrating keratoplasties after herpetic infection. Transplants were done in healthy eyes using homologous and autologous tissue, and once the grafts were well healed, they were infected with herpes simplex at various times after keratoplasty. Allografts and autografts behaved similarly: Ten days after infection they developed epithelial and superficial stromal disease with vascularization. Eventually, most grafts partially cleared after the inflammatory process subsided, but some allografts and autografts remained opaque and vascularized without ever demonstrating a typical rejection pattern. Histologically, the cells present in the opaque graft were lymphocytes and plasma cells, which are also found in graft rejections. They concluded that in this type of experiment, graft rejection due to tissue incompatibility was not induced by the herpetic infection. Rice and Jones had found, however, that in their series,[12] graft rejections were more frequent in patients with herpetic keratitis. The experimental study mentioned above does not deny these authors' observations, since what seems to be crucial is the preexistence of corneal vessels and lymphatics in the host tissue. Even though reference is only made to vessels and not to lymphatics, which I consider important,[13] Maumenee,[14] Fine and Stein,[4] and Khodadoust[3] have unquestionably shown that host vascularization increases the incidence of graft reactions; therefore, this may be one of the most important factors to consider when we talk about causes of graft failure. Size of graft, reaction to suture material, and uveitis are other factors that may stimulate the development of graft rejection in patients with chronic herpetic disease. In addition to these conditions, percolation or transport of herpes simplex virus (HSV) antigens from host to graft may occur. This tissue is then sensitized and behaves as a new antigenic source.

Of more interest than the actual fate of grafts infected with HSV, is the question of virus persistence in the stroma of grafts obtained from donors with previous herpetic disease. Polack et al.[15] performed penetrating grafts in rabbits using convalescent (well healed) corneas. A number of grafts opacified and later partially cleared, while others remained opaque and vascularized. Epithelial disease was never seen in these convalescent grafts, but the stromal opacities showed accumulations of lymphocytes and plasma cells around degenerated keratocytes. When examined with the electron microscope, these areas failed to show the presence of HSV; however, the cellular reaction was similar to that seen in cases of experimental graft reaction. Unquestionably, these studies cannot be equated with clinical situations because, in the rabbit, graft rejections occur rarely in the first set of grafts in contrast to rejection in human eyes in which rejections occur in at least 10% of grafts done in favorable cases. It is well known also that eyes with chronic keratitis are usually vascularized and, therefore, present a potential risk for an immune reaction increasing the chance of rejection to 20%–30%. In another series of experiments, we investigated the behavior of corneal tissue (grafts), previously infected or exposed to herpes antigens, placed in animals that had been systemically or locally sensitized to HSV.[16] Even though no virus could be cultured or found in previously infected grafts, these showed HSV fluorescein-labeled antigens in the stroma and were rapidly destroyed by massive infiltrations of round cells and vessels. The rejection occurred within 2 wk after grafting and showed no typical pattern of graft rejection, but rather rapid clouding and vascularization like that seen in xenograft rejections. The rejections were more violent in animals that had been locally sensitized. When grafts from animals systemically sensitized to HSV were placed in eyes locally sensitized (intracorneal), 50% of them developed clouding in an accelerated fashion, indicating that viral antigens had reached the cornea of the donor animal.

Similar, but less defined, results were obtained in experiments where the host and donor had been systemically or locally sensitized to streptococcal antigens.[17] Both types of experiments indicate that foreign proteins, particularly those from common viruses and bacteria, may modify the host immune system and anatomical structure of recipient sites. In this way, second-set-like reactions may arise when grafts sensitized to common antigens are given to recipients sensitized to similar antigens.

HERPETIC KERATITIS AND KERATOPLASTY IN HUMANS—CLINICAL OBSERVATIONS

Since herpetic keratitis varies in extension and severity in most cases, evaluation of clinical results of keratoplasty requires an adequate classification, because results may vary according to the stage and extension of the process. A classification such as that of Hogan et al.[18] is conveniently systematized and describes a clinicopathologic picture that helps to determine the site and extension of the process (Table 13-3). It is obvious that one stage of the disease may extend or overlap into another one; however, this basic scheme is very practical and didactic, and it has been used to classify our cases undergoing keratoplasty.

Antivirals and steroids[19] have modified, to some extent, the course of chronic herpetic keratitis in a large number of patients; however, they have not prevented the development of corneal scarring or reduced the frequency of recurrences. As previously mentioned, the problem of herpetic keratitis lies not only in the area, or areas, where the virus exists or proliferates, but also in the more complex problem of tissue sensitization to herpetic antigens.[19] Graft failure in HSV-infected hosts, therefore, can be traced not only to viral reinfection, but also to an immune response to HSV antigens. As mentioned above, it can also be due to intraocular or external inflammation, and to an immune response to transplantation antigens (graft reaction). In our experiments, it became evident that anti-herpes antibodies in sensitized hosts can rapidly destroy HSV-sensitized grafts. Possibly the same type of immune reaction is present in HSV-infected

Table 13-3
Classification of Herpetic Keratitis

I.	Superficial
	1. Dendritic keratitis without stromal involvement
	2. Dendritic keratitis with stromal involvement
	3. Geographic epithelial keratitis (late superficial)
II.	Deep
	1. Stromal keratitis without ulceration (disciform)
	2. Healed stromal leukoma
	3. Stromal keratitis with ulceration
	A. Nonperforating
	B. Perforating
III.	Keratouveitis
	1. Uveitis with keratitis
	A. Without ulceration
	B. With ulceration
IV.	Postherpetic keratopathy (metaherpetic)

Reproduced by permission.[18]

host corneas, and the disease can be cured in some cases by removing the diseased tissue. If this is true, the larger the graft, the less the chance for recurrence or inflammation, since most of the diseased tissue was removed. But we must remember that the closer a graft is to the limbus, the better the chance for an immune reaction. Therefore, here we have a situation where the size of the graft becomes a very important item and possibly the type of sutures used. The excellent results published by Rice and Jones[12] in active herpetic keratitis treated by penetrating keratoplasties tend to support this concept, which is not discussed in their paper. These authors obtained 77% clear, penetrating grafts in cases of active herpetic keratitis and 79% in inactive cases. Even though 57.9% of these grafts had edema postoperatively, they cleared on steroids, and only 8.8% developed recurrences. In our series of 26 cases, there were 20 active keratitis cases and 6 inactive. All of the inactive cases remained clear as compared to only 45% of the active cases. In spite of steroid and antiviral treatment, our recurrence rate was 75%.[11] Other authors[4,9] have reported around 60% of clear grafts with 24%–40% incidences of recurrences. They found that intensive use of topical steroids reduced the incidence of recurrences from a previous level of 84% in nongrafted eyes.[9] Pfister et al.[20] had only two grafts done in the acute stage in a series of 28 penetrating keratoplasties, and both failed. Their over-all failure rate in this series was 53%, and their failure rate with lamellar grafts was 57%. Lamellar or penetrating keratoplasty has been recommended for herpetic keratitis; however, it is agreed that either form of keratoplasty in active cases should be avoided if possible until the eye quiets down. In our experience and that of others, lamellar keratoplasty has a worse prognosis in active or vascularized corneas. Steroids can stimulate virus replication in the most unusual way in situations where its use appears to be indicated.[21] When analyzing keratoplasty results from different authors, it is difficult to obtain a simple answer in this area because of the variations in severity and extension of the corneal disease as well as the immune response of the host.

It is apparent that herpetic antigens can persist in the host and appear in the graft that may succumb to an immune reaction (tissue incompatibility or HSV response). However, active viral replication can exist in some grafts with recurrences, as shown by Dawson et al.[22] and Collin and Abelson.[21]

REFERENCES

1. Castroviejo R: Selection of patients for keratoplasty. Surv Ophthalmol 2:1–12, 1958
2. Castroviejo R: Atlas de Queratectomias y Queratoplastias. Barcelona, Salvat, 1964
3. Khodadoust AA: The allograft reaction: The leading cause of late failure of clinical corneal grafts, *In* Porter R, Knight J (eds): Corneal Graft Failure. Ciba Foundation Symposium, New York, Elsevier, Excerpta Medica, North-Holland, 1973, pp 151–167
4. Fine M, Stein M: The role of corneal vascularization in human allograft reactions. *In* Porter R, Knight J (eds): Corneal Graft Failure. Ciba Foundation Symposium. New York, Elsevier, Excerpta Medica, North-Holland, 1973, pp 193–208
5. Polack FM: Clinical and pathologic aspects of the corneal graft reaction. Trans Am Acad Ophthalmol 77:418–431, 1973
6. Gibbs DC, Batchelor JR, Casey TA: The influence of HLA compatibility on the fate of corneal grafts, In Porter R, Knight J (eds): Corneal Graft Failure. Ciba Foundation Symposium. New York, Elsevier, Excerpta Medica, North-Holland, 1973, pp 293–306
7. Paton D: The prognosis of penetrating keratoplasty based upon corneal morphology. Ophthal Surg 7:36–45, 1976
8. Stuart JC, Mund MC, Iwamoto T, et al: Recurrent granular corneal dystrophy. Arch Ophthalmol 79:18–24, 1975
9. Moore TE, Aronson SB: The corneal graft: A multiple variable analysis of the penetrating keratoplasty. Am J Ophthalmol 72:205, 1971
10. Polack FM, Wind C, West C: The fate of experimental corneal grafts in herpetic keratitis and keratouveitis. Invest Ophthalmol 14:917–922, 1975
11. Polack FM, Kaufman HE: Keratoplasty in herpetic keratitis. Am J Ophthalmol 73:908–913, 1972
12. Rice N, Jones B: Problems of corneal grafting in herpetic keratitis, *In* Porter R, Knight J (eds): Corneal Graft Failure. Ciba Foundation Symposium. New York, Elsevier, Excerpta Medica, North-Holland, 1973, pp 221–239
13. Polack FM: *In* Maumenee AE: Discussion of clinical patterns of corneal graft failure, *In* Porter R, Knight J (eds): Corneal Graft Failure. Ciba Foundation Symposium. New York, Elsevier, Excerpta Medica, North-Holland, 1973, pp 15–22
14. Maumenee AE: Clinical pattern of corneal graft failure, *In* Porter R, Knight J (eds): Corneal Graft Failure. Ciba Foundation Symposium. New York, Elsevier, Excerpta Medica, North-Holland, 1973, pp 5–15
15. Polack FM, Hawa MH, Valenti J, et al: Ultramicroscopic changes in corneal graft after HSV sensitization. (in preparation)
16. Polack FM, Siverio C, Bigar F, et al: Immune host response to corneal grafts sensitized to herpes simplex virus. Invest Ophthalmol 3:188–195, 1976
17. Vidal R, Polack FM: Denevir des keratoplasties experimentales apres sensibilisation par un antigene bacterien. (streptocoque groupe A). Arch Ophthalmol (Paris) 36:765, 1976
18. Hogan MJ, Kimura SJ, Thygeson P: Pathology of herpes simplex kerato-iritis. Trans Am Ophthalmol Soc 61:75–99, 1963
19. Bachellor JR: Grafting in herpetic keratitis, *In*: Porter R, Knight J (eds) Corneal Graft Failure. Ciba Foundation Symposium. New York, Elsevier, Excerpta Medica, North-Holland, 1973, p 235

20. Pfister RR, Richards JS, Dohlman C: Recurrence of herpetic keratitis in corneal grafts. Am J Ophthalmol 73:192, 1972
21. Collin H, Abelson M: Herpes simplex virus in human cornea, retrocorneal membrane, and vitreous. Arch Ophthalmol 94:1726–1729, 1976
22. Dawson C, Togni B, Moore T: Structural changes in chronic herpetic keratitis: Studies by light and electron microscopy. Arch Ophthalmol 79:740–747, 1968
23. Salleras A: Bullous keratopathy, *In* King J, McTigue J (eds): The Cornea World Congress. Washington, Butterworths, 1965, pp 292–299

Chapter 14

Pathology of the Corneal Graft

To a great extent, results of keratoplasty are fairly predictable if the factors mentioned in previous chapters are taken into account—particularly our knowledge of donor tissue characteristics, its functional potential after grafting, and the background host disease. It is true that to this date we have not solved the biologic problem of graft rejection, but we can minimize the causes of mechanical problems that favor the immune reaction. Knowing that the donor tissue is very delicate has led us to improve our techniques in tissue handling, instrumentation, sutures, etc. There are, however, a series of complications that may eventually cause opacification of the graft. Some of them can be prevented (lid closure defects, trichiasis, entropion, dry eye, glaucoma, iritis), while others are truly unexpected immediate or later complications (infections, wound rupture, hemorrhage). Primary donor tissue failure is a preventable complication, but it may occur when tissue of borderline viability is used, even if the donor had been a young adult and the cornea used within 24 hr. This has been observed with donor eyes from alcoholics, cachectics, or patients with long agonies. Occasionally, our methods of examining donor eyes cannot detect functionally inadequate tissue.

Causes of graft failure will be discussed in this chapter with emphasis on clinical and pathologic findings and methods of prevention or treatment. The immune graft reaction will be dealt with in a separate chapter.

DONOR TISSUE FAILURE

In our discussion of donor tissue viability, as it relates to age of the donor and time of storage, we came to the conclusion that older donor tissue with many hours of storage (more than 20 hr) was not ideal donor material, because its endothelial layer has a decreased number of cells when compared to young adult corneas.[1-4] However meticulous the surgical technique, there is an unavoidable loss of a certain number of endothelial cells during keratoplasty, particularly in phakic grafts.[5-7] These investigators have shown that up to 80% cell loss can occur without affecting the transparency of the graft or its corneal thickness measurements. It is also known that a large number of endothelial cells can be lost from grafts cut with scissors, as compared to grafts cut from the endothelial side with a trephine.[8] In contrast to animal corneas, which may heal primarily by endothelial cell division, human endothelial cells heal areas of damage by enlarging their cell body, as has been shown by specular microscopy in corneas after intraocular surgery.[5,7,9] The endothelium of the donor cornea may not be able to

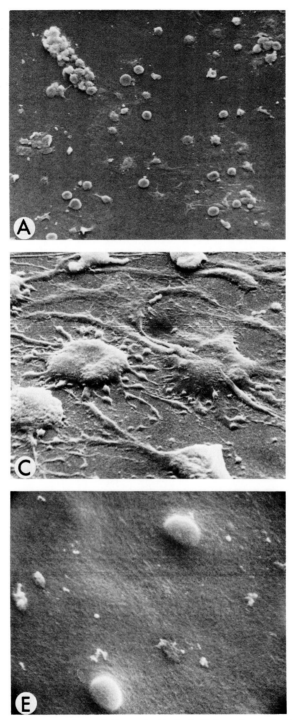

Figure 14-1. Donor tissue failure. **A.** Endothelial surface of a failed graft showing Descemet's membrane almost completely devoid of endothelial cells. Clumps of inflammatory cells are attached to Descemet's membrane (SEM, ×100). **B.** At higher magnification, this picture shows enlarged endothelial cells surrounded by leukocytes (SEM ×500). (Reproduced by permission.[37]) **C.** Several dead endothelial cells covering normal Descemet's membrane in a failed cryopreserved graft (SEM, ×1000). (Repro-

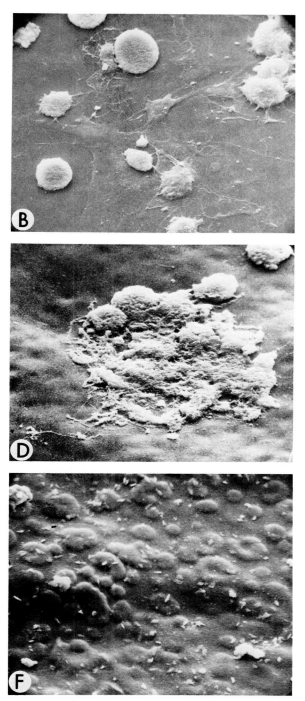

duced by permission.[37]) **D.** Another case of failed donor tissue showing
Descemet's membrane covered by clumps of destroyed endothelial cells
and leukocytes (SEM, ×500). **E.** Descemet's membrane of a failed graft
showing abnormal surface with two warts and absence of endothelial cells
(SEM, ×2000). **F.** Descemet's membrane of another failed graft showing
multiple warts and few endothelial cells. Debris contaminates the endothelial surface (SEM, ×500).

cover Descemet's membrane if the loss of endothelial cells at the time of surgery was great and the number of cells is below 500/sq mm. In this case, the graft will opacify. This situation is more critical if the donor tissue has an abnormal Descemet's membrane (Fuchs' dystrophy), which, in the absence of warts, may pass unnoticed through the slit-lamp screening. When vitreous appears in the anterior chamber after surgery, it tends to adhere to areas of abnormal graft endothelium or to interfere with endothelial regeneration and function. Grafts with adherent vitreous may become cloudy rapidly or remain semitransparent for several weeks and then gradually increase in thickness and eventually opacify. This depends on the degree of endothelial trauma and its regenerative ability, as well as the structure of the vitreous. Opaque corneal grafts (due to tissue failure), removed within a week after keratoplasty, have been examined with the scanning electron microscope. They show large flat endothelial cells with numerous cytoplasmic prolongations partially covering a smooth, normal Descemet's membrane or clumps of rounded, dead endothelial cells (Figs. 14-1 **A–D**). Other grafts show no endothelium, but a Descemet's membrane with a spongy irregular surface (Fig. 14-1**E**) or multiple warts typical of Fuchs' dystrophy (Fig. 14-1**F**), indicating that in these two cases, tissue failure was related to Fuchs' dystrophy in the donor eye.

Graft edema occurring 24 hr after surgery, which in spite of treatment (steroids, control of elevated intraocular pressure, hypertonic saline solution) gets worse (0.9 mm–1.0 mm.) in 2 days, usually indicates irreversible tissue failure. It has been our preference to replace the cloudy graft as soon as the diagnosis of tissue failure has been made. In phakic cases, we may wait 1 or 2 wk if the host cornea has normal endothelium (keratoconus). In these cases, serial pachymetry may show slow but progressive thinning.

Improperly handled cryopreserved tissue may suffer total or partial detachment of the endothelial cell layer (Fig. 14-2**A**). Often, cell loss is not always related to surgical trauma or tissue with low viability, but to the presence of early dystrophic changes (Fig. 14-2**B**). Fibrous metaplasia with permanent Descemet's membrane folds are found in grafts with edema persisting for many weeks. These fibrotic changes are more conspicuous in failed tissue with vitreous adhesion in a localized spot (Figs. 14-2 **C,D**), where membranes and fibrocytes are found, not necessarily from endothelial origin (Fig. 14-2**E**). Failed grafts with diffuse vitreous contact (observed personally at the time of surgery) show multiple areas of abnormal, absent, or destroyed endothelium with fibrous membrane formation (Fig. 14-2**F**).

WOUND LEAK, WOUND DEHISCENCE, AND WOUND RUPTURE

Since the microscope was introduced in corneal surgery and small sutures became available, wound closure has not been a major technical problem in keratoplasty. Leakage through suture tracts may occur in eyes with severe scarring and thinning due to chemical burns or bacterial infection, particularly those

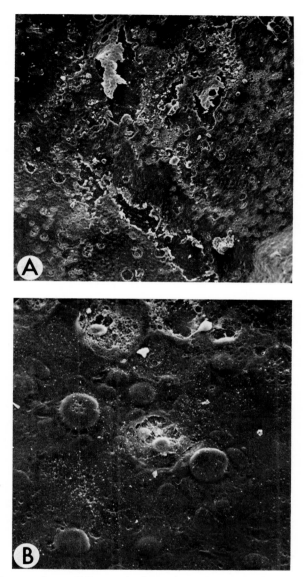

Figure 14-2. Donor tissue failure. **A.** Scanning electron microphotograph of the endothelial surface of a cryo-preserved cornea. The specimen shows large areas of endothelial abrasion that appear to be artifactual. The endothelial layer, however, shows multiple isolate or confluent lesions, which vary between 9 and 20 μ in diameter (SEM, ×100). **B.** An area of the previous picture showing endothelial cells surrounded by warts, some of which are very prominent. Rounded lesions correspond to the destruction of the cell membrane of one or more endothelial cells (SEM, ×720).

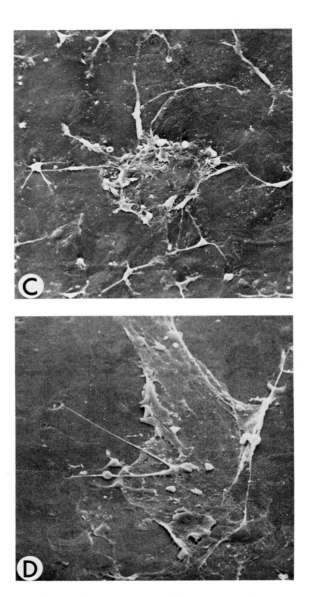

C. Failed corneal graft due to vitreous contact. The electron microphotograph shows one area of vitreous adhesion with absence of endothelial cells and fibrous reaction. Fibroblastic cells are present over the abnormal endothelial layer (SEM, ×440). **D.** Appearance of the endothelial surface of another failed graft with vitreous contact. The graft endothelium shows multiple areas of vitreous adhesion to areas devoid of endothelial cells or fibrous strands attaching to Descemet's membrane (SEM, ×1000).

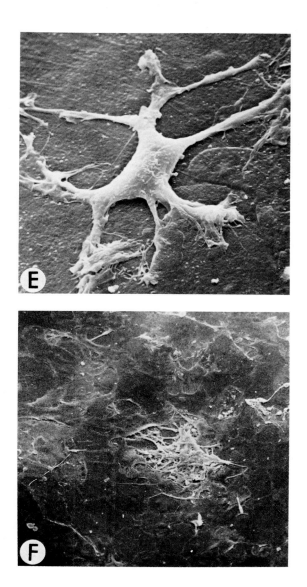

E. Fibroblast-like cell frequently observed in cases of vitreo-corneal adhesion. This cell straddles endothelial cells to the right and an abnormal Descemet's membrane to the left (SEM, ×3200). **F.** Endothelial surface of a failed graft of long-standing. The picture shows a large area of vitreous adhesion with fibroblastic reaction and endothelial cell alterations consistent with retrocorneal membrane formation (SEM, ×500).

due to Pseudomonas. In contrast to normal corneas where stromal swelling closes the suture track, in scarred corneas, filtering of aqueous humor may occur around deeply placed 10'0' monofilament nylon because of the thickness disproportion between the suture and the needle. Another reason is that because of its elasticity, nylon must be tied with extra force, possibly resulting in widening of the needle tract.

Shallowing or flattening of the anterior chamber 24 hr or more following surgery may be due to leakage around a defectively placed suture and/or to pupillary block if the intraocular pressure is elevated; however, it may be associated with choroidal detachment and low pressure. If the glaucoma does not respond to oral glycerol (1 g/kg) or intravenous mannitol (1 g/kg) therapy, a peripheral iridectomy should be performed.

Early wound separation (weeks) due to prolonged use of topical steroids or sub-Tenon's injections of deposteroids has been observed while sutures are in place and may be associated with structural changes in host and graft tissue ("melting"). This complication is often associated with or preceded by ectasia of the graft and increased intraocular pressure. Extrusion of nylon or silk sutures with gaping of the wound is corrected by resuturing with 8'0' black or virgin silk, taking large bites; discontinuing steroids; and, in some cases, using a bandage contact lens. If glaucoma has been present, it should be well controlled.

Late wound dehiscence (6–10 mo or longer) usually occurs as a result of trauma or premature removal of sutures, and it is often related to the frequent use of topical steroids. Only experience can tell when a corneal incision appears properly healed before the sutures are removed. This complication is more frequent in cases of severe corneal edema in which the graft was sutured with nylon. Deep vessels in the scar indicate adequate healing most of the time, but in edematous corneas, healing is slow even with vessels in the scar. In these corneas, I prefer to suture the graft with 9'0' silk (Ethicon 1702, GS-8) or 8'0' virgin silk material (Ethicon 1736, GS-9; Davis and Geck, CE-30) in order to stimulate rapid healing. In cases where 10'0' running nylon has been used, Kaufman[10] recommends a second continuous suture of 13μ nylon, which is left in place permanently (Chapter 12, Fig. 12-6).

Complete wound rupture with sudden loss of the anterior chamber has a poor prognosis if the graft rapidly becomes edematous. This indicates rupture or detachment of Descemet's membrane, and it is frequently due to trauma shortly after suture removal[11] (Figs. 14-3**A,B**). Folds in Descemet's membrane rapidly become surrounded by fibroblastic cells (Figs. 14-3**C,D**) and become permanent. In cases of long-standing edema, a fibrous membrane covers the abnormal Descemet's membrane (Figs. 14-3**E,F**). In Moore and Aronson's series,[21] wound ruptures occurred 5½ yr after keratoplasty following trauma or after 1 yr following herpetic or bacterial infection at the host–graft junction. The massive infiltration by leukocytes in cases of inflammation may cause lysis of collagen that is preferentially arranged in a circular fashion (see chapter 10). Most likely, Descemet's membrane has not fully regenerated in these cases.

Choroidal detachment is often associated with perforated corneas or ruptured wounds. Rodriguez-Barrios (personal communication, 1975) advises choroidal taps when repairing these wounds.

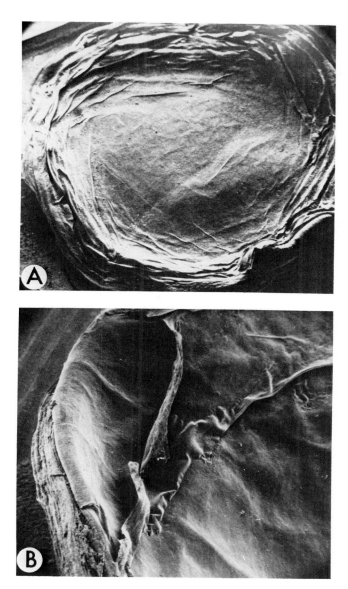

Figure 14-3. **A.** Scanning electron microphotograph of a failed graft following wound dehiscence. The graft shows partial detachment of Descemet's membrane at the periphery with multiple formation of folds (SEM, ×20). **B.** Photograph showing a torn Descemet's membrane following traumatic rupture of the wound (SEM, ×50).

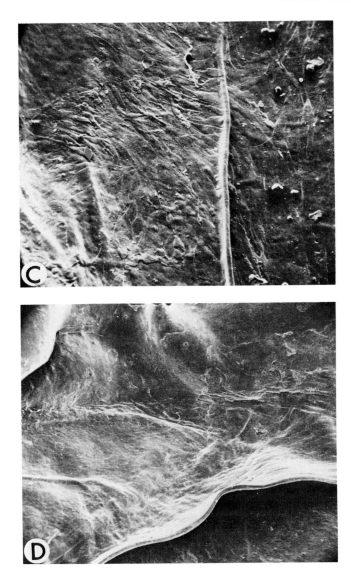

C. The appearance of a small fold in Descemet's membrane in a case of recent wound dehiscence. The fold is surrounded by elongated endothelial cells with evidence of fibroblastic metaplasia (SEM, ×100). **D.** The photograph shows the torn edge of Descemet's membrane in a graft with wound rupture. Absence of endothelial cells and fibroblastic activity are characteristic findings in injured Descemet's membrane (SEM, ×100).

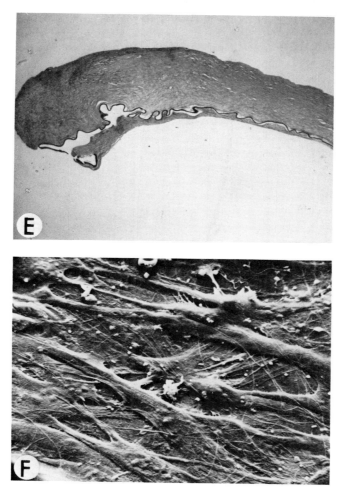

E. Cross-section of a failed graft due to wound rupture. Multiple Descemet's membrane folds are present in the periphery of the graft, which is thickened and covered by a thick retrocorneal membrane (hematoxylin and eosin, ×50). **F.** Picture showing the fibroblastic activity over Descemet's membrane in cases of corneal edema of long-standing following wound rupture (SEM, ×500).

GRAFT ULCERATION

Incomplete healing of graft epithelium is sometimes seen in eyes with previous grafts, abnormal conjunctival tissue (chemical burns), and deficient tear film. It is likely to occur in transplants in which the donor epithelium was removed by scalpel scraping "in order to reduce the amount of antigenic material." This method of getting rid of donor epithelium is no longer recommended;[12] instead, a very light rubbing of the surface with a gauze or wet cellulose sponge should be done to eliminate cell debris and leave an intact basement membrane. If epithelial ulceration is not detected early or not given enough attention, a deeper ulceration is sure to develop with compromise of the graft transparency. This problem may also occur, perhaps with more frequency, in lamellar grafts with preserved or frozen tissue.

Provided that no frequent topical medication is required, small epithelial defects usually heal with a firm dressing left in place undisturbed for 48–72 hr. Removal of the dressing should be followed by frequent instillations of methylcellulose drops or artificial tears during the daytime and a plain ophthalmic ointment at bedtime. If there is evidence of epithelial edema, hypertonic saline drops should be used instead of artificial tears.

In cases where medication is to be given frequently (antibiotics, steroids, cycloplegics, etc.), a bandage soft lens is the treatment of choice.[13] In central defects, which are the ones most frequently seen, a Softcon lens[14,15] or a B-L bandage lens can be left in place for several weeks if it is adequately fitted.

While collagenolytic enzymes may play an important role in slow healing epithelial defects, in general, we have not required the use of collagenase inhibitors as others have recommended.[16,17] Hypertonic saline solution can be used in grafts with epithelial edema associated with these erosions.

Epithelial ulcerations in the lower portion of the graft are usually related to bulky sutures, defective lid closure, entropion, or trichiasis. The immediate treatment is that of a bandage soft lens; subsequently, repair of the lid anomaly may be performed. Occasionally, one sees minor epithelial defects due to abnormal tear film or filamentary keratitis, which respond well to bandaging with a soft contact lens. Epithelial lesions may become infected with fungus or bacteria causing deep ulcers and irreversible damage to the grafted tissue (Figs. 14-4**A,B**). Even without perforation, the endothelium underlying the ulcer will be covered by inflammatory cells, fibrin, fibroblasts, and pigment granules (Figs. 14-4**C,D**). In failed grafts after infection has subsided, few normal endothelial cells may be found over Descemet's layer.

GRAFT VASCULARIZATION

In contrast to superficial corneal vascularization, deep host corneal stromal vascularization is one of the major risks for the development of graft rejection. This clinical fact was known even before the mechanism of graft reaction was well understood, but it has been demonstrated experimentally[18] and in large clinical series.[19,20] It was also shown by Moore and Aronson[21] that silk sutures

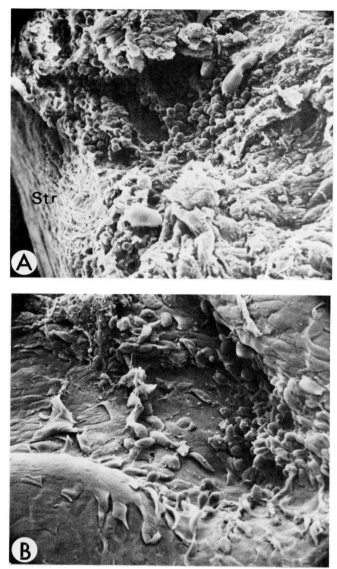

Figure 14-4. Graft ulceration. **A.** Scanning electron microphotograph of a deep ulceration in a graft. The ulcerated area is filled with debris and inflammatory cells and compromises the deep stroma (Str, stroma; SEM, ×500). **B.** A more superficial corneal graft ulceration showing desquamated and dead epithelial cells as well as some leukocytes (SEM, ×50).

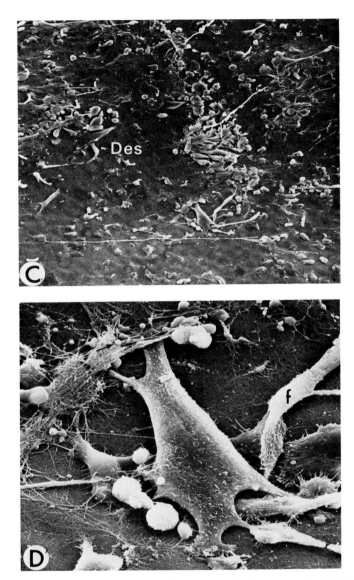

C. Endothelial surface of a graft with a deep corneal ulceration (aphakic). Descemet's membrane (Des) is devoid of endothelial cells centrally. Macrophages, fibroblasts, and inflammatory cells form nodular formations on its surface. Other endothelial cells are abnormal and partially cover Descemet's membrane (SEM, ×500). **D.** A large macrophage, fibroblast-like cells (f), leukocytes, and fibril strands with pigment granules (arrow) are found over a bare Descemet's membrane (SEM, ×3000).

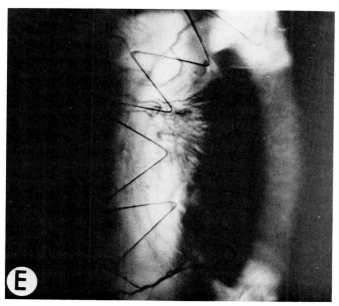

E. Penetrating graft sutured with 10'0' nylon. New vessels follow sutures.

tend to aggravate or to induce greater stromal vascularization. Even though monofilament nylon sutures may induce vascularization[24] (Fig. 14-4**E**), they are the ideal materials for suturing grafts with vascularized corneas. In these recipient eyes, any preexisting condition that may be causing inflammation of the anterior segment must be eliminated. Particular attention should be given to chronic blepharitis or iritis, and moderate use of steroids may be necessary to quiet the red eye. Three conditions, however, should be given special consideration before and after keratoplasty, because they need a different therapeutic approach based on the disease background, severity, and natural course. These are: rosacea keratitis, herpetic keratitis, and keratitis in Stevens-Johnson's syndrome. At our institution, the use of beta irradiation prior to keratoplasty is rather limited, mostly because of wound-healing complications.

HERPETIC INFECTION

Results of penetrating keratoplasty in herpetic keratitis vary according to the stage and activity of the disease.[22,23,25] Grafts done in active herpetic keratitis usually have a high incidence of reactivations (see chapter 15) or failure due to inflammation.

Herpetic graft infection usually starts at the host–graft junction as a deep epithelial ulcer, and it usually takes an irregular geographic aspect. Although virus cultures have always been negative in these ulcers, they should be treated as active herpetic disease with topical antivirals. Recent concepts[26,27] indicate that

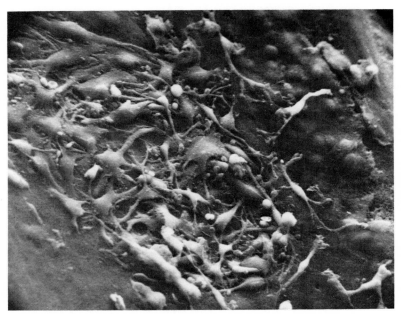

Figure 14-5. Herpes infection. Granulomatous reaction on Descemet's membrane in a case of recurrent herpetic keratitis. Giant cells, fibroblasts, leukocytes, and pigment granules are present (SEM, ×500). (Reproduced by permission[37])

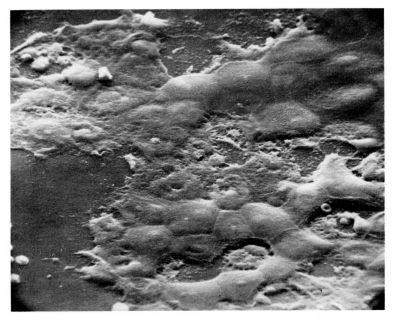

Figure 14-6. Herpes infection. An area of endothelial cell destruction in herpetic keratitis (SEM, ×500).

this type of epithelial–stromal disease has an immunologic basis that can be modified with the simultaneous use of topical steroids. Failed grafts, due to herpetic inflammation, show stromal infiltration with round cells and areas of collagen destruction. Deep stromal compromise may cause granulomatous reactions in Descemet's membrane (Fig. 14-5). Stromal disease is usually associated with uveitis and a concomitant destruction of endothelial cells (Fig. 14-6).

GLAUCOMA

Post-keratoplasty glaucoma may develop in phakic eyes as a result of pupillary block, fibrinous iritis, peripheral synechiae, or following flattening of the anterior chamber due to defective wound closure. In aphakic eyes, transient glaucoma is present in over 50% of cases without operative complications or inflammation of the anterior segment. The etiology has not been elucidated, but it is probably related to blockage of outflow channels by vitreous components, anatomical changes in outflow channels, or obliteration of the meshwork due to lack of Decemet's membrane support, as suggested by D. Willard (personal communication, 1975). In most cases, it resolves within a few weeks (this would support transient blockage), but in others, treatment is needed for several months.

Measurement of intraocular pressure in eyes with edematous corneas or corneas with irregular surfaces, as we find in most transplants, can be obtained with the MacKay-Marg tonometer, as shown by Irvine et al.[28] or one of the applanation air tonometers. Even though the mires of the Goldman applanation tonometer can be observed relatively well in grafts of large size, measurements tend to be much lower than the actual pressure. Often, the Schiotz tonometer will give values closer to the MacKay-Marg instrument in cases of elevated intraocular pressure (J. Buxton, personal communication, 1975).

In aphakic patients, carbonic anhydrase inhibitors are used immediately after surgery, even if the intraocular pressure was normal before transplantation. If the pressure remains below 20 mm Hg 2–3 days after surgery, the drug is discontinued, but the pressure should be monitored daily. If, in spite of Diamox or Neptazane, the intraocular pressure appears elevated, glycerol (1 g/kg) is given orally, two to three times a day. We prefer to delay the use of miotics as long as possible in cases of postoperative elevated intraocular pressure in aphakia; but, they should be started if the pressure remains high after 2 or 3 days on hyperosmotic agents and carbonic anhydrase inhibitors because of the risk of electrolyte imbalance. Even in the absence of peripheral synechiae, many aphakic patients will show persistent elevated intraocular pressure that will require long-term antiglaucoma therapy.

Elevated intraocular pressure should be suspected in patients with phakic grafts if ocular pain occurs or if diffuse graft edema develops. In these eyes, the angle is not visible because of the suture line or because the peripheral host cornea is cloudy; therefore, judging the depth of the anterior chamber is not a satisfactory way to determine angle compromise. Frequently, one finds that graft thickness is normal or reduced in the presence of high intraocular pressure, and thickness may suddenly increase when the pressure is normalized.

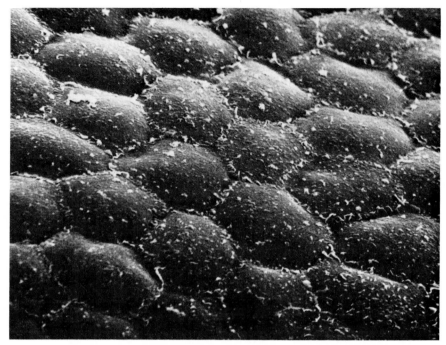

Figure 14-7.   Glaucoma. A moderate degree of endothelial cell edema in an experimental graft with induced glaucoma (SEM, ×2000).

In experimental grafts of eyes with increased pressure, there is cell edema (Fig. 14-7), stretching of endothelial cell junctions, and cell death. Since human endothelium has a limited regenerative ability, failed grafts with glaucoma show few fibroblast-like endothelial cells or cells of large size (Fig. 14-8). In other cases, we have observed fibrous membranes in totally opaque grafts. It was apparent in our studies in rabbits and those of Svedbergh[28] in monkeys that moderate intraocular pressure elevations for periods of a few hours may cause severe endothelial cell damage. Cell swelling is perhaps the earliest lesion, followed by vacuolization, cell junction rupture, blebbing, plasma membrane rupture, and cell death. Svedbergh postulates that in chronic glaucoma, cells may heal areas of destruction. Increase in cell size would be found in these late stages. In the late postoperative period, peripheral synechiae and pupillary block are the most common causes of elevated intraocular pressure in the absence of anterior segment inflammation. Steroid-induced glaucoma may be the cause if the drug had been used for several weeks; therefore, steroids must be discontinued.

Persistent elevated intraocular pressure in spite of medical therapy may require surgical control. In aphakic eyes, our treatment of choice has been cyclocryotherapy[29] and, occasionally, subscleral sclerectomy. These procedures, however, may cause opacification of recent grafts and are reserved for old grafts as a last resort.

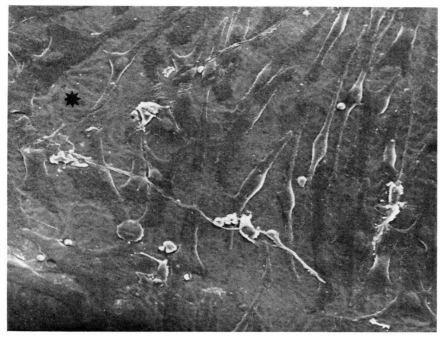

Figure 14-8. Glaucoma. The endothelium of a corneal graft with glaucoma of long-standing. There are some large endothelial cells, areas of Descemet's membrane without cell covering (*), and several fibroblast-like endothelial cells (SEM, ×1000).

ANTERIOR CHAMBER HEMORRHAGE

A small hyphema in the anterior chamber of phakic eyes immediately after transplantation usually reabsorbs without compromise of the graft transparency. In some instances, the elevated intraocular pressure associated with the hyphema may require the use of hyperosmotic agents in order to protect the wound and to prevent damage to the corneal endothelium. Hyphema is of more severe consequence when associated with fibrinous iritis or in aphakic eyes. In these two circumstances, it tends to reabsorb very slowly and often becomes organized behind the graft, forming a peculiar retrocorneal membrane (Figs. 14-9 and 14-10). The hemorrhage may change from red to brown and eventually turn grey-white in subsequent months. This is due to loss of hematic pigment from red cells that can be identified in histologic preparations several months later at the time of regrafting. In cases of hyphema due to iritis in aphakic or phakic eyes, any attempt to remove this by lavage of the anterior chamber is usually unsuccessful and only induces additional irritation of the iris and increases the risk of more synechiae and endothelial destruction. However, in cases of hyphema due to bleeding from deep stromal vessels or from the iridectomy at the time of surgery, it is possible to remove this material by anterior chamber

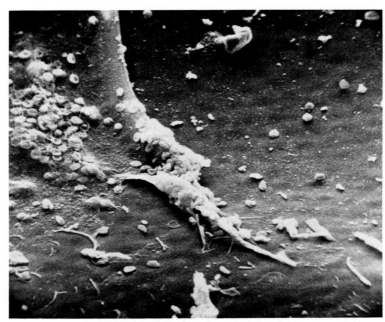

Figure 14-9. Anterior chamber hemorrhage. Scanning electron microphotograph of the endothelial surface of a failed corneal graft with anterior chamber hemorrhage. A thick white membrane covers most of the central portion of the graft. Areas around this membrane are devoid of endothelial cells (SEM, ×20). (Reproduced by permission.[37])

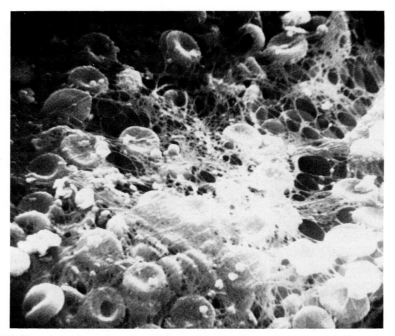

Figure 14-10. Anterior chamber hemorrhage. Microphotograph of a retrocorneal membrane in a case of anterior chamber hemorrhage. This membrane is composed of fibrin, old red blood cells, and pigment granules (SEM, ×1000). (Reproduced by permission.[37])

irrigation in phakic eyes or before it becomes organized in aphakic eyes by the use of a vitreous cutting instrument through the pars plana. At this institution, good results have been obtained with the Girard-Sparta phacofragmentor, the Machemer VISC, and the Douvas rotoextractor. These patients should have careful control of their intraocular pressure as well as systemic and topical use of steroids. It can be said that the prognosis is usually poor when hyphema occurs in a fresh graft. I agree 100% with Fine[30] who considers the endothelium of a recent corneal graft equivalent to the endothelium of a cornea with early dystrophy.

SYNECHIA AND POSTERIOR GRAFT MEMBRANES

As is well known, the risk of peripheral synechia increases with the diameter of the transplant. In eyes where iritis is suspected or has been present, it is important to minimize this complication by the use of topical and systemic steroids several days before surgery. In aphakic eyes or in eyes where a graft and lens extraction were performed simultaneously, the risk of synechia to the wound may increase if an incomplete vitrectomy was performed or if vitreous fibrils on the wound appear connected with the iris, forming synechiae to the pupillary border or to the mid-iris. There is clinical and experimental evidence that any iris synechia to the wound will predispose the eye to graft reaction;[31] however, in most cases, the risk of causing endothelial damage and graft clouding while attempting lysis of these adhesions is higher than that of an immune reaction. Synechiae of less than one quadrant, which are not progressing in the course of 2–3 wk should be left alone; however, if these synechiae progress along the wound edge in several days of follow-up, it is important to separate them from the graft and restore the chamber with balanced salt solution or Miochol (acetylcholine), if pupillary constriction seems necessary. Lysis of synechia is performed with a Castroviejo 0.5-mm spatula through a Ziegler knife incision in the quadrant opposite to the synechia. Synechiae can be lysed as early as 10 days after keratoplasty, but a delay of many weeks may result in their organization, and at the time of lysis, a detachment of graft Descemet's membrane may result, particularly if the sweep is toward the graft instead of along the length of the wound. Unfortunately, in the areas of iris adhesions, the endothelium is replaced by fibrous tissue (Fig. 14-11). In patients with vitreous or iris adhesions, it is important to determine if the peripheral iridectomy is open and if a partial pupillary block is bound to develop by organized vitreous. In some of these patients, we have performed one or two peripheral laser iridectomies.

Vitreous adherent to the wound may not present problems for a long time, but eventually, these bands become thicker and connective tissue spreads around and over the graft, causing endothelial cell metaplasia and graft opacification. Management of vitreous is of utmost importance at the time of aphakic keratoplasty where a careful anterior vitrectomy is indicated. Because of the high incidence of macular edema associated with this type of vitrectomy, we now prefer to do extracapsular cataract extraction when these are required in combination with keratoplasty. Release of vitreous adhesion in late postoperative periods usually requires an anterior vitrectomy, which should be done before the

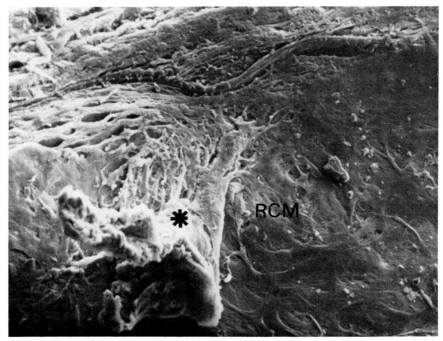

Figure 14-11.   Scanning electron microphotograph of the edge of a failed graft with iris synechiae (*). Endothelial cells near this adhesion have formed a retrocorneal membrane (RCM) (SEM, ×2000).

vitreous becomes organized. Even so, grafts with a low number of endothelial cells may not survive this procedure.

Retrograft membranes are a common finding in rejected grafts and also in failed grafts due to nonviable donor tissue, wound rupture, inflammation, etc. Grafts placed within the membrane of a previously failed graft are likely to be covered by the scar tissue, unless the new graft is of larger size and is done through an area free of fibrous proliferation.

GRAFT FAILURE DUE TO NONSPECIFIC INFLAMMATION

Ocular inflammation has been indicated as another cause of graft opacification,[32,33] especially in avascular corneas. Experiments were performed[34] to exclude graft opacification as a result of tissue sensitization. To this effect, we performed autografts and allografts in rabbits, and when they were well-healed, an immunogenic uveitis was induced[35] by intravitreal injection of bovine serum albumen (BSA).[36] The intraocular inflammation caused transient opacification of allografts and autografts, thus excluding transplantation immunity as a cause of graft cloudiness. Moore and Aronson[21] induced similar reversible graft opacification by systemic BSA sensitization in grafted rabbits and subsequent challenge with topical BSA administration (allografts and autografts). In chapter 5, we have mentioned experiments where grafts could also opacify, due to immune response to herpetic or bacterial antigens.

Clinically, it is difficult to prove these situations, but they must be considered since they may coexist or precede a tissue immune reaction. Perhaps herpetic uveitis is the most frequent cause of this type of opacification, but chronic bacterial infections of sinuses or teeth are also conditions that deserve prompt attention. In experimental situations, graft cloudiness is reversible because the endothelium of rabbit corneas regenerates rapidly. Human endothelium does not have this potential, and anterior chamber inflammation may cause irreparable damage to this layer through antigen–antibody complexes, leukotoxins, lysozymes, etc.

REFERENCES

1. Irvine AR, Irvine AR Jr: Variations in normal human corneal endothelium. Am J Ophthalmol 36:1272–1285, 1953
2. Kaufman HE, Capella, JA, Robbins JE: The human corneal endothelium. Am J Ophthalmol 61:835–841, 1966
3. Laing RA, Sandstrom M, Berrospi AR, et al: Changes in the corneal endothelium as a function of age. Exp Eye Res 22:587, 1976
4. Bourne WM, Kaufman HE: Specular microscopy of human corneal endothelium in vivo. Am J Ophthalmol 81:319–323, 1976
5. Bourne WM, Kaufman HE: Clinical specular microscopy of the corneal endothelium, In Kaufman HE, Zimmerman TJ (eds): Current Concepts in Ophthalmology vol 5. St. Louis, C.V. Mosby, 1976, pp 264–271
6. Bourne WM, Kaufman HE: The endothelium of clear corneal transplants. Arch Ophthalmol 94:1730, 1976
7. Laing RA, Sandstrom M, Berrospi AR, et al: Morphological changes in corneal endothelial cells after penetrating keratoplasty. Am J Ophthalmol 82:459, 1976
8. Brightbill F, Polack FM, Slappey T: A comparison of two methods for cutting donor corneal buttons. Am J Ophthalmol 75:3, 1973
9. Forstot SL, Blackwell WL, Jaffe NS, et al: The effect of intraocular lens implantation on the corneal endothelium. Trans Am Acad Ophthalmol Otolaryngol 83:195–203, 1977
10. Kaufman HE: Combined keratoplasty and cataract extraction. Am J Ophthalmol 77:824, 1974
11. Polack FM, Binder PS: Detachment of Descemet's membrane from grafts following wound separation: Light and scanning electron microscopic study. Ann Ophthalmol 7:47, 1975
12. Jones BJ: Introduction to the problem of corneal graft failure, In Porter R, Knight J (eds): Corneal Graft Failure. Ciba Foundation Symposium. New York, Elsevier, Excerpta Medica, North-Holland, 1973, p 1
13. Kaufman HE, Uotila MH, Gasset AR, et al: Medical uses of soft contact lenses, In Gasset AR, Kaufman HE (eds): Soft Contact Lens. St. Louis, C.V. Mosby, 1972, p 175
14. Gasset AR: Griffin Naturalens (bandage lens) in treatment of bullous keratopathy, dry eyes, and corneal ulcers, In Gasset AR, Kaufman HE (eds): Soft Contact Lens. St. Louis, C.V. Mosby, 1972, p 210
15. Shaw EL, Aquavella JV: Anatomical and physiological basis of contact lens fitting. Contact Lens J 2:53, 1976

16. Dohlman C: The function of the corneal epithelium in health and disease. Invest Ophthalmol 10:383, 1971

17. Brown S, Hook C: Treatment of corneal destruction with collagenase inhibitors. Trans Am Acad Ophthalmol Otolaryngol 75:119, 1971

18. Polack FM: Histopathological and histochemical alterations in the early stages of corneal graft rejection. J Exp Med 116:709, 1962

19. Khodadoust A: The allograft rejection reaction: The leading cause of late failure of clinical corneal grafts. In Porter R, Knight J (eds): Corneal Graft Failure. CIBA Foundation Symposium. New York, Elsevier, pp 151, 1973

20. Fine M, Stein M: The role of corneal vascularization in human corneal graft reaction, In: Corneal Graft Failure. CIBA Foundation Symposium. New York, Elsevier, Excerpta Medica, North-Holland, 1973

21. Moore T, Aronson S: The corneal graft—A multiple variable analysis of the penetrating keratoplasty. Am J Ophthalmol 72:205, 1971

22. Polack FM, Kaufman HE: Penetrating keratoplasty in herpetic keratitis. Am J Ophthalmol 73:908, 1973

23. Pfister RR, Richards JS, Dohlman CH: Recurrence of herpetic keratitis in corneal grafts. Am J Ophthalmol 73:192, 1972

24. Fine M, Jones S: The role of corneal vascularization in human corneal graft reaction: Discussion, In Porter R, Knight J (eds): Corneal Graft Failure. CIBA Foundation Symposium. New York, Elsevier, Excerpta Medica, North-Holland, 1973, p 207

25. Rice N, Jones B: Problems of corneal grafting in herpetic keratitis, In Porter R, Knight J (eds): Corneal Graft Failure. CIBA Foundation Symposium. New York, Elsevier, Excerpta Medica, North-Holland, 1973, p 221

26. Kaufman HE: Herpetic stromal disease, Editorial. Am J Ophthalmol 80:1092, 1975

27. Metcalf JF, Kaufman HE: Herpetic stromal keratitis: Evidence for cell-mediated immunopathogenesis. Am J Ophthalmol 82:827, 1976

28. Irvine A: Measurement of intraocular pressure after penetrating keratoplasty, In Polack FM (ed): Corneal and External Disease of the Eye. Springfield, Ill, Charles C Thomas, 1970, pp 353–358

29. Svedbergh B: Effects of artificial intraocular pressure elevation on the corneal endothelium in the vervet monkey. Acta Ophthalmol 53:938, 1975

30. West CE, Wood TO, Kaufman HE: Cyclocryotherapy for glaucoma pre or post-penetrating keratoplasty. Am J Ophthalmol 76:485, 1973

31. Fine M: Problems of keratoplasty in aphakic eyes, In Dabezies OH, Gitter KA, Samson CLM (eds): Symposium on the Cornea, Transactions of the New Orleans Academy of Ophthalmology. St. Louis, C.V. Mosby, 1972, p 143

32. Polack FM: Clinical and pathological aspects of the corneal graft rejection. Trans Am Acad Ophthalmol Otolaryngol 77:418, 1973

33. Castroviejo R: Cornea and Lens Symposium: Ocular Allergy. Trans Am Acad Ophthalmol Otolaryngol 56:242, 1952

34. Castroviejo R: Atlas de Queratectomias y Queratoplastias. Barcelona, Salvat, 1969

35. Polack FM: The effect of ocular inflammation on corneal grafts. Am J Ophthalmol 60:259, 1965

36. Silverstein AM, Zimmerman LE: Immunogenic endopthalmitis produced in the guinea pig by different pathogenic mechanisms. Am J Ophthalmol 48:435, 1961

37. Polack FM: The endothelium of failed corneal grafts. Am J Ophthalmol 79:251, 1975

Chapter 15

The Corneal Graft Reaction

Technically successful corneal transplants in avascular corneas usually heal without any impairment of the transparency of the graft and remain clear for indefinite periods of time. It has been shown that this tolerance to a homograft is not due to lack of antigenicity of the donor cornea or to an absence of lymphatic channels in the host, but to its avascular character (see chapter 6). In this respect, it is well known to the clinician that the prognosis for functional results of corneal grafts in vascularized corneas is almost always fair to poor[1-10] unless the graft is modified by corticosteroids or HLA-matched. Even so, many of these grafts opacify as a result of an immune reaction.[11]

In some ways, the corneal graft rejection can be compared to the rejection of a skin graft that is destroyed by leukocytes and eventually is replaced by fibrous tissue. This tissue destruction, which occurs with other transplanted organs as well, develops after a period of host sensitization. It is well known, however, that in contrast to skin grafts, which become necrotic and are eliminated after rejection, the rejection of corneal grafts does not follow the same fate. Even though scarring following rejection can be permanent, in many instances, the degree of opacification can be lessened by early and adequate treatment with corticosteroids or immunosuppressive drugs.

The rejection of corneal grafts is a manifestation of delayed hypersensitivity, similar to that induced by viral, bacterial, or heterologous protein antigens. There is now ample evidence to show that it is in the lymphatic tissue that antibodies in general and those specifically responsible for graft rejection are formed.[12-14] We showed, in 1965,[15] that the morphological response to xenografts and also allografts involves the lymphatic tissue present in the ocular tissues (bulbar and palpebral conjunctiva, orbital tissue), systemic lymphoid tissues, the reticulo-endothelial system, and the graft itself.

The morphological changes in the corneal graft can be best studied in the experimental animal, where the early stages of the immune rejection can be examined at the light and ultramicroscopic levels. These early changes have provided insight into the complex phenomenon of full-thickness graft rejection and factors that influence its development.

THE IMMUNE CORNEAL GRAFT REJECTION IN MAN

In 1948, Paufique, Sourdille, and Offret[16] used the term "maladie du greffon" (graft sickness) to describe the phenomenon of graft opacification for which no clinical explanation could be found. According to them, this reaction occurred 10 days after grafting and was an allergic manifestation to the transplanted tissue. They also described another group of patients in which graft cloudiness developed in the third postoperative week, this being interpreted as a disturbance in the metabolism of the graft. Mueller and Maumenee[17] stated that if the nature of the "graft sickness" was allergic, it would occur later than 10 days postoperatively and would correspond to the "third-week opacification" of the French authors. Before the third week it is not possible, on a clinical basis, to distinguish an immunoallergic graft reaction from graft opacification due to postoperative complications. Graft rejection rarely occurs before the third week. A period of graft transparency before the development of opacification is then a requirement in making the clinical diagnosis of graft reaction, since no diagnostic laboratory test is available. The graft reaction usually occurs a few months (3–5 mo) after transplantation, but can appear several years later. Sometimes, minor corneal trauma or ocular inflammation has precipitated the immune reaction.

Clinical Picture

The rejection of a penetrating corneal graft can start at the level of the epithelium, stroma, or endothelium, separately or in two or three layers at once.[11-18] Epithelial rejection, however, often passes unnoticed because it occurs in an inconspicuous fashion, often in a mildly inflamed eye, and this reaction must be looked for carefully.[18] The most frequent type of rejection occurs in the endothelium (Fig. 15-1**A** and **B**), and it might be preceded by redness of the conjunctiva and circumcorneal vascular engorgement. Two forms of rejection usually occur: (1) diffuse graft edema with scattered keratitic precipitates (KPs), a mild aqueous flare and edema of the posterior layers of the graft; and (2) graft edema, which begins near the scar, usually near the area of vessel ingrowth, defective wound healing, or iris synechiae. In one-third to one-half of the cases, a band of white cells will be prominently deposited between the normal corneal endothelium and the opaque (rejected) area at the periphery of the graft. These precipitates, which mark the edge of the rejected endothelium, were shown in 1962 and 1964 in flat endothelial preparations from experimental corneal grafts[8-19] and were also demonstrated later in rabbits by Khodadoust and Silverstein,[29] who called them a "rejection line." Today, it is considered the only pathognomonic evidence of an immune graft rejection,[18] since such distribution of KPs and pattern of opacification is not observed in any other disease. This focal and progressive type of rejection can be accompanied by aqueous flare and iritis and by prominent engorgement of host stromal vessels.[11] More rarely, a severe edema with whitening of the graft may occur almost overnight, suggesting rapid destruction of the endothelium.

Persistent graft edema due to iritis, glaucoma, or wound defects will stimulate the growth of vessels into the stroma of the graft, which will be eventually rejected and replaced by scar tissue. According to Maumenee,[2] the severity of the immune reaction is usually inversely proportional to the length of time that the transplant has been clear, a viewpoint shared by others.

Postoperatively, it is not enough to establish the clarity of a graft, but edema must be detected before clinical signs of rejection appear. Very early graft thickening can be determined by pachymetry, and the progress of the disease as

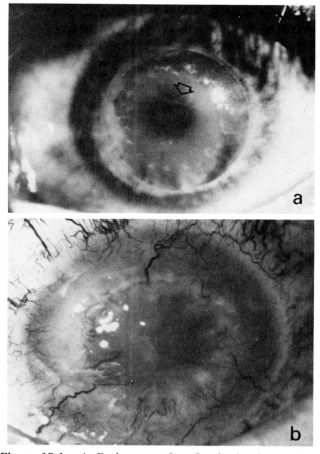

Figure 15-1. **A.** Early stage of graft rejection in a patient with keratoconus. There is diffuse graft edema and a line of keratic precipitates (arrow) that have moved from the scar toward the center of the graft. **B.** Advanced stage of graft rejection with stromal opacification and vascular invasion. Usually endothelial rejection precedes this stage.

well as its response to steroids can be followed closely (Fig. 15-2). The recipient cornea, if avascular, remains clear during the rejection process.

Lamellar allografts may also induce an immune reaction when placed in a vascular bed; their rejection, however, is not as frequent as that of penetrating transplants. In my experience, the rejection of lamellar transplants has occurred more frequently in large (9.5 or 10 mm) and thick grafts, usually performed for keratoconus. These large grafts usually require careful follow-up and long-term (months) topical steroid therapy to avoid rejection. The clinical picture of lamellar graft rejection is characterized by engorgement of limbal vessels with vascular invasion of the graft stroma (Fig. 15-3); occasionally, vessels may also grow between the graft and the recipient cornea. Epithelial rejection may be observed more frequently with large lamellar grafts than with penetrating transplants,

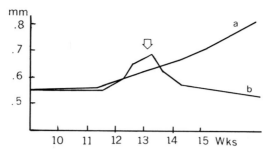

Figure 15-2. Diagram showing graft thickness measurements in two cases. **A.** Rejection started 11 wk post-keratoplasty, and rejection progressed to total opacification due to inadequate therapy. **B.** Therapy was started with topical steroids as soon as the thickness increased. Rejection was reversed 1 wk later with systemic steroids (arrow).

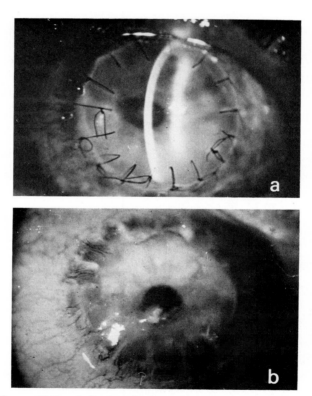

Figure 15-3. **A.** Early rejection of a 9-mm lamellar graft 4 wk after keratoplasty. A previously clear graft is now hazy. There is ciliary congestion and infiltration around sutures. Removal of sutures is necessary at this time. **B.** Rejection of a lamellar graft 2 mo after keratoplasty. Sequential epithelial defect appears to be rejection of epithelium. Vessels are encroaching on the stroma of the graft.

perhaps because of their large size in contrast to the smaller size of penetrating keratoplasties.

In some instances, an early graft rejection (less than 1 mo after keratoplasty) may occur in the second lamellar or penetrating graft when the time lapse between the first and second transplants has been of a few months. Even though homologous tissue from different donors should not induce an accelerated type of rejection, tissue antigens of similar structure may be shared by corneal cells to the extent that antigenic stimulation by some shared antigens is enough to induce a full graft rejection.[21,22] The rejection of xenografts is due to sensitization to serum proteins as well as to tissue antigens.

EXPERIMENTAL GRAFT REJECTION

Penetrating corneal allografts in clear avascular rabbit corneas are not usually rejected. However, a small number of grafts, 5%–10%[23] (less than 5% in my experience) will spontaneously reject after vascularization has occurred.

When the transplants are done in vascularized host corneas, 10%–20% will opacify after a period of transparency. Corneal grafts in rabbits with normal corneas are rejected regularly if a skin graft from the corneal donor is also done at the time of corneal surgery or even later (second-set rejection). In our experiments, we have grafted approximately 1 sq in of skin 2 wk after corneal grafting to those animals with clear, well-incorporated grafts,[1] thus eliminating cloudy grafts due to technical problems. A period of sensitization, which varied from 12

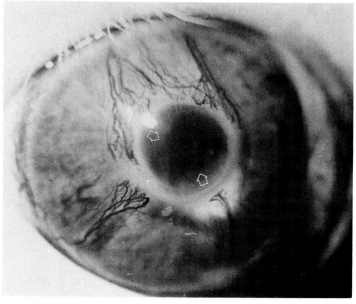

Figure 15-4. Endothelial rejection developed in two areas of a clear experimental graft (arrows). New vessels are filling the scar in these areas and begin to invade the stroma superiorly.

to 16 days, preceded the beginning of graft opacification. In most cases, a crescent-shaped area of corneal edema was observed in the periphery of the graft after engorged deep limbal vessels reached the scar.[8] The edema was always in the area of vessel ingrowth (Fig. 15-4) and could appear simultaneously in one or more places when more than one set of vessels surrounded the transplant. Usually, the cloudy area was neatly separated from the normal graft, and in many cases, a line of white cells (KPs) was present between these two areas that is similar to the rejection line seen in humans. Total opacification and vascularization usually occurred in 5–7 days.

Skin grafting produces a situation previously described and known as a "second-set phenomenon." This reaction is known to be more severe than the reaction to a first homograft; but the clinical and the histopathologic pictures are identical to that seen in humans.

THE REACTION OF THE LYMPHATIC TISSUES

It is assumed that histocompatibility antigens travel by way of lymphatic channels to the regional lymph nodes, from where the process of sensitization proceeds throughout the lymphoid system (Fig. 15-5). Little is known, however, about how or in what form the antigens leave the graft, but it is believed that cells can release antigenic particles without being destroyed and reform them again on its plasma membrane. Except at the limbus, the cornea lacks lymphatic channels to transport such antigens, but this function may very well be carried out by the interfibrilar and interlamellar spaces, as suggested in experiments described in chapter 6. Vascularized corneas with newly formed lymphatic channels have the potential of carrying antigens faster or in greater amount than avascular corneas. We know for example, that allografts in vascularized corneas (interstitial keratitis) may have an early and severe rejection.

Before intralamellar corneal xenografts are invaded by round cells and vessels, morphological changes are present in the regional lymph nodes, spleen, and liver.[15] These observations favor the theory of sensitization by way of

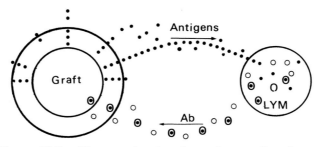

Figure 15-5. Diagram showing the pathways of graft antigenic sensitization (black dots) and antibodies bound to cells (circled black dots) or free (clear circles). Antibodies may reach the graft from its surface, through the host stroma, or through the anterior chamber.

lymphatic channels, in contrast to the other possibility, mentioned by Medawar,[24] that the inductive phase of graft rejection is initiated in the graft itself. This theory would require lymphocytes from the blood to reach the graft, react with antigens, and then travel back to the lymph nodes where the effector cells would be generated.

Systemic study of the lymphatic tissue has not been made in animals with rejected corneal homografts after skin grafts, because such changes could have been produced by the skin graft and not by the corneal graft itself. However, even in cases where the skin graft was placed in the abdomen, a notable hyperplasia of the subconjunctival lymphatic tissue at the beginning of the homograft rejection (Fig. 15-6), as well as round-cell infiltration of the limbus of the grafted eye (Fig. 15-7), was observed. During the rejection process, lymphocytes are present in the different corneal layers, but at the limbus, they appear between endothelial vascular cells and their connective tissue sheath. These have the appearance of newly formed lymphocytes, suggesting in situ replication (Fig. 15-8). The limbal origin of immunocompetent lymphocytes has been pointed out by Elliott et al.,[25] Parks et al.,[26] and Howes.[27] This latter author showed ferritin-labeled lymphocytes in the limbal area of rabbits with immunoallergic keratitis. In most of our experiments with homografts, we have seen accumulations or clumps of small lymphocytes and some plasma cells. The small lymphocyte has been identified tentatively as the "immunologically competent" cell responsible for the graft reaction.[28] Although there is evidence that antibodies may cause cell destruction,[18] it seems that direct contact between activated lymphocytes and donor cells is necessary for their destruction. It is possible that anticorneal antibodies in the aqueous humor might cause endothelial damage and graft

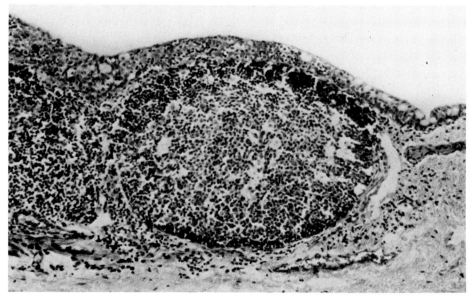

Figure 15-6. Hyperplasia of lymphoid conjunctival tissue of an experimental graft at the time of rejection (hematoxylin and eosin, ×10).

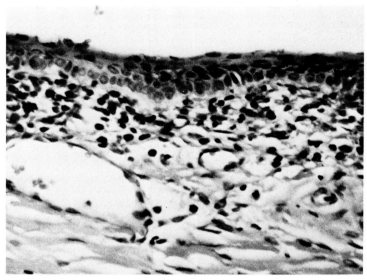

Figure 15-7. Hyperplasia of subconjunctival limbal lymphoid tissue in a rabbit eye with graft rejection (hematoxylin and eosin, ×10).

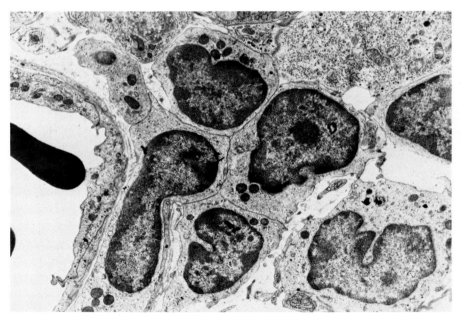

Figure 15-8. Several lymphocytes around a limbal capillary in a rabbit eye with graft rejection. These cells have large nuclei with dense chromatin granules, the cytoplasm has prominent mitochondria, and cells are in the process of division (×6000). (Reproduced by permission.[42])

opacification,[29] but sensitized lymphocytes originating in the uvea may cause diffuse cell damage,[30] a situation demonstrated experimentally by Silverstein and Khodadoust[31] with passively transferred lymphocytes to the anterior chamber of rabbit eyes.

MATERIALS AND METHODS

Penetrating corneal grafts were made in albino rabbits, as described previously[8] (chapter 1.). Eyes were examined daily with a slit lamp 1 wk after skin grafting and were removed for histologic study at different stages of the graft reaction. Tissues were prepared for light microscopy after being fixed in 10% formalin. Carnoy-fixed grafts were used for flat endothelial preparations. Tissue for transmission and scanning electron microscopy were fixed in 2.5% or 4% buffered glutaraldehyde as described below.

Histology

LIGHT MICROSCOPY

Flat endothelial mounts of corneas fixed in Carnoy's solution for 24 hr were prepared. Descemet's membrane and the endothelium of the host and graft were removed in one layer under the operating microscope; the specimen was mounted on a gelatin-coated slide and stained with hematoxylin and eosin. Flat tangential sections of the remaining stroma[8] were cut with a freezing microtome and stained with Harris' hematoxylin and eosin. Frozen sections, cut tangentially to the surface, were also made from grafted corneas fixed in 8% formalin for 5 days or longer, and stained with toluidine blue (pH 4.5) for metachromasia.

SCANNING ELECTRON MICROSCOPY (SEM)

The corneas of eyes bearing corneal grafts in various stages of rejection were bathed with drops of cooled 2.5% or 4% glutaraldehyde. At this point, the animals that had been kept under anesthesia were killed by an additional injection of sodium pentobarbital, the eyes were removed, and the corneas carefully excised. The tissue was immersed in cold glutaraldehyde, where they were fixed for 8–12 hr, then rinsed in phosphate buffer and post-fixed in 1% osmium tetroxide for 1 hr. The tissue was then cut into smaller pieces and dehydrated in graded series of alcohols. Final samples were dried in a critical-point apparatus (Bomar) or freeze-dried. Dried samples were mounted on aluminum stubs with conductive paint, coated with gold palladium, and examined in a scanning electron microscope (Stereoscan-Cambridge, Zeiss, or Jeol). The samples were studied at either 10 or 20 kV, and pictures were taken with Polaroid P/N film.

TRANSMISSION ELECTRON MICROSCOPY (TEM)

As previously, the cornea was fixed while the animal was under anesthesia. The rabbit was killed, the eye removed, the cornea excised and immediately fixed in 1% osmium tetroxide buffered with 0.15 M sodium cacodylate, pH 7.4, at 4°C for 1 hr. It was then dehydrated rapidly through graded series of alcohols;

while in 80% ethanol, the pieces were cut in 1–2-mm blocks and embedded in Epon 812 after infiltration with propylene oxide. One to two micron sections were stained with azure-2 or toluidine blue for light microscopy. Thin sections were cut with glass or diamond knives on a Porter-Blum ultramicrotome, mounted on palladium-coated copper meshes double-stained with uranil and lead citrate, and examined in a Siemmens Elmiscope 1 or in a Zeiss electron microscope.

RESULTS

Morphological alterations in the rejected graft will be described at the levels of (1) scar tissue, (2) epithelium, (3) stroma, and (4) endothelium. Changes in the ground substance were demonstrated by a metachromatic stain and the uptake of radioactive sulfate. The study was done in over 100 rabbit allografts.

Scar Tissue

The scar is more a component of the host than of the graft,[31–33] but it is an area of considerable importance in graft rejection. Histologic studies of healing scars in normal corneal grafts reveal that this is a most active area of regeneration in the first few days after surgery. Several weeks after the operation, the proliferation of connective tissue in the normal scar decreases gradually; several months later it may be reduced to a thin line in which collagen fibers tend to fuse with the pattern of normal corneal fibers.[34] (see chapter 4).

After blood vessels reach the wound, the scar tissue appears swollen under the slit lamp microscope. Histologic observations of cross-sections of the grafted cornea show the scar infiltrated by large and small lymphocytes, plasma cells, and a small number of polymorphonuclear leukocytes. The vessels that reached the scar usually do so through the anterior or middle third of the cornea (Fig. 15-9).

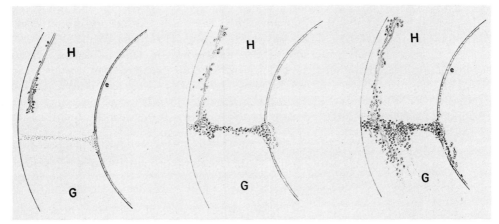

Figure 15-9. Diagram showing the pattern of deep corneal vascularization and graft invasion by vessels and white cells. Lymphocytes and plasma cells invade the scar and reach the anterior chamber through the unhealed Descemet's membrane at the host–graft junction.

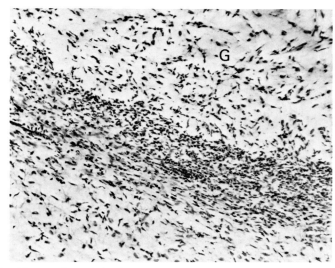

Figure 15-10. Flat section of the host–graft junction showing the scar during the rejection process. This area is infiltrated by lymphocytes and plasma cells (G, graft; hematoxylin and eosin, ×100).

This cellular infiltration reaches Descemet's endothelium simultaneously or before invading the stroma of the graft. Flat frozen sections revealed cellular infiltration of the scar, which was more severe in the vascularized areas (Fig. 15-10). Newly formed vessels at the host–graft junction spread out in a brush-like fashion, forming a fine network that eventually penetrates the graft. With the electron microscope, the tips of these vessels show budding processes and alignment of endothelial cells with a small narrow lumen present towards the blind capillary end (Figs. 15-11 and 15-12). The appearance of these vessels is

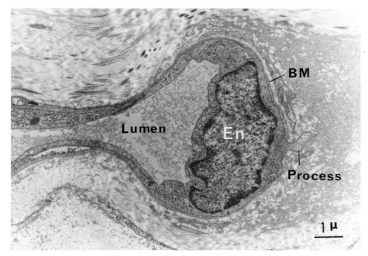

Figure 15-11. Tip of a new vessel in a vascularized cornea. It shows a budding process in a vascular endothelial cell (En). Basement membrane (BM) is present (TEM, ×10,000). (Reproduced by permission.[43])

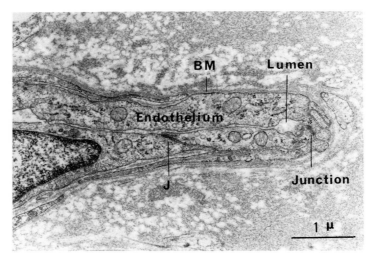

Figure 15-12. Another area of vascularized cornea showing the end of a vessel where two endothelial cells form a tight junction while leaving a small lumen (BM, basement membrane; J, junction; TEM, ×23,000). (Reproduced by permission.[43])

the same in the scar tissue and in the rejected graft stroma. Vessels were surrounded by lymphocytes that reached the posterior surface of the scar and eventually entered the anterior chamber through Descemet's membrane. This structure was not yet regenerated across the wound; (Figs. 15-13 and 15-14) instead, the wound showed a bridge of thick collagen tissue. Cells present in the protruding scar tissue were fibroblasts, monocytes, lymphocytes, and plasma cells; some of these advanced towards the graft endothelium, which began to show cell destruction near the scar (Fig. 15-15). This inflammatory process was more prominent in the graft side of the scar. Scanning electron microscopic studies of the scar, in early rejection stages, showed a beginning of lymphocytic infiltration of graft endothelium and the progression of these cells toward the peripheral endothelial layer (Fig. 15-16**A, B** and **C**). Grafts with poor coaptation

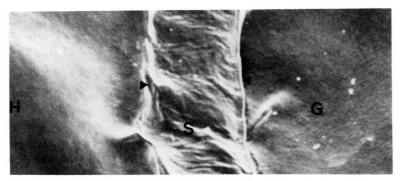

Figure 15-13. Scanning electron microphotograph of the host–graft junction of a 4-wk-old graft with normal apposition showing the edges (arrows) of cut Descemet's membrane (H, host; G, graft; S, scar; SEM, ×100).

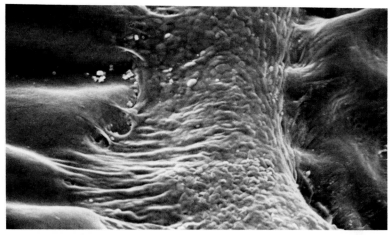

Figure 15-14. The host–graft junction of a 4-wk-old graft with prominent scar tissue at the beginning of rejection. Occasional lymphocytes are over the scar (SEM, ×200).

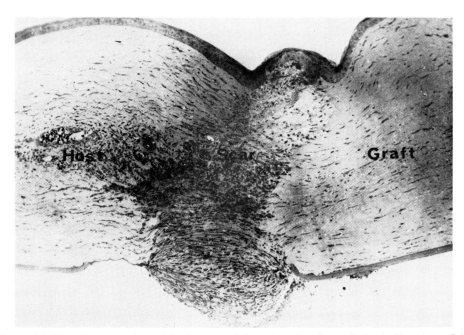

Figure 15-15. Cross-section of the host–graft junction showing cellular infiltration of the scar with round cells penetrating the anterior chamber and invading the graft endothelium (×130). (Reproduced by permission.[44])

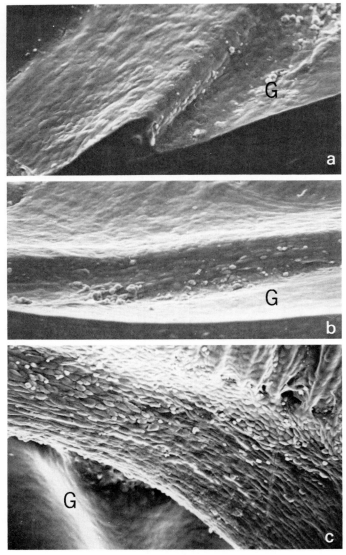

Figure 15-16. Scanning electron microphotographs of the host–graft junction at the beginning of the rejection process. **A** and **B** show round cells entering the anterior chamber through or between endothelial cells. **C** shows a slightly more advanced infiltration of the scar. Leukocytes advance only towards the graft (G, graft; SEM, ×100, ×100, and ×500, respectively).

show an abundance of scar tissue and a large degree of infiltration; the amount of scar tissue present in several grafts varied and was related to the type of cut and approximation afforded by the sutures. It appeared that thicker scars would swell more and have more vessels and more infiltration by white cells.

Epithelium

The rejection of graft epithelium is characterized by a linear irregularity in the graft surface that can be detected with a vital dye, such as methylene blue or Congo red. Fluorescein lightly stains the affected epithelium because only a few cells are destroyed at one time, as can be seen in Figure 15-17. With the scanning electron microscope, disorganization of the corneal epithelial mosaic is apparent around a line of destroyed cells, pits, or craters. The edges of these narrow lines sometimes show elevations or lumps that correspond to lymphocytes present in the subepithelial layer (Fig. 15-18). Examination of the rejected area under high-power magnification shows destroyed epithelial cells on the graft side of the rejection line and large cells with prominent microvilli on the host side of the rejection line. Possibly, these cells corresponded to host cells migrating across the transplant behind the rejection line.

When the rejected epithelial area was examined in plastic-embedded sections stained with toluidine blue, basal epithelial cells were present on either side of the rejection line. They appeared flattened, rectangular or triangular in shape. The rejected cells weakly stained with toluidine blue, whereas host cells stained normally. In the central portion of the rejection line, epithelial cells

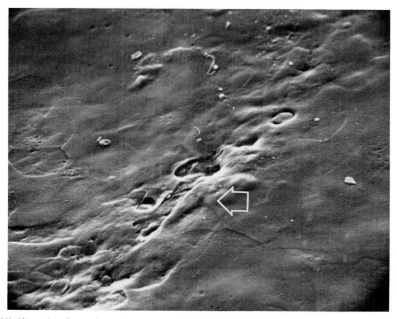

Figure 15-17.   Graft surface showing epithelial rejection that advances in the direction of the arrow. Some of the superficial cells are absent. In other areas, subepithelial lymphocytes form lumps on the surface (SEM, ×500).

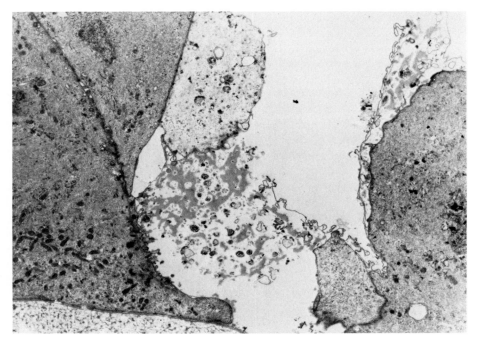

Figure 15-18. Section of corneal graft epithelium at the level of the line of rejection shown in Figure 15-17 (TEM, ×4200). (Reproduced by permission.[45])

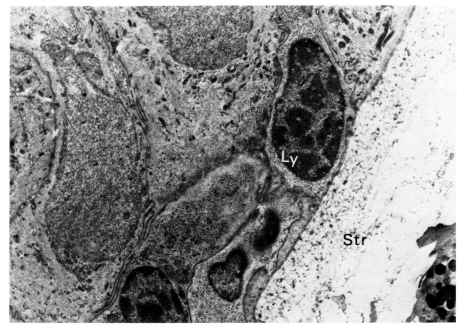

Figure 15-19. Two lymphocytes (Ly) in the basal epithelial layer. These cells enter the epithelium through the basement layer and move towards the surface (Str, stroma; TEM, ×3400).

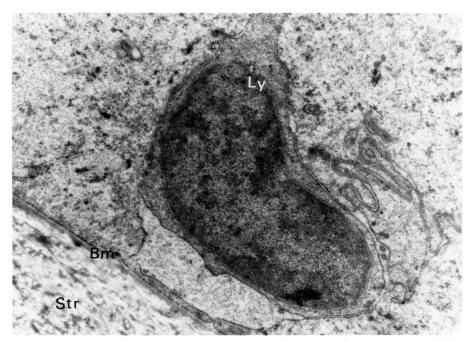

Figure 15-20. A small lymphocyte (Ly) has gained access to the basal epithelial layer between two epithelial cells during a graft rejection episode. (Str, stroma; BM, basement membrane; TEM, ×10,000).

showed rupture of their plasma membrane and disorganization of their cytoplasmic structure (Fig. 15-18). In some sections, only the remaining plasma membrane attached to the basement membrane could be observed; while in others with simultaneous stromal rejection, there was a destruction of the basement epithelial membrane that was invaded by macrophages. Lymphocytes were present between the epithelial cell layers mostly in the basal layer (Fig. 15-19). The cytoplasmic cellular interdigitation was altered at the site of lymphocyte contact, resulting in a smooth cell boundary without desmosomes. In most areas, the epithelial cells in contact with lymphocytes showed cytoplasmic vacuolization and lysosomes. Those lymphocytes present within the rejected epithelial cell layer were smaller than epithelial cells, round-, oval-, or pear-shaped with round or oval nuclei and a condensed chromatin (Fig. 15-20). They contained mitochondria, sparse endoplasmic reticulum, a Golgi complex, and free ribonucleoprotein (RNP) granules. There were no plasma cells in the areas of epithelial cell rejection.

Stroma

Morphological changes present in keratocytes varied in different grafts and in different lamellae. Cell changes were characterized by retraction of corneal cell processes and elongation of nuclei and cytoplasm. In general, graft changes were related to the presence of vessels in the stroma and these seem to follow endothelial cell alterations and corneal edema. Monocytes, lymphocytes, plasma

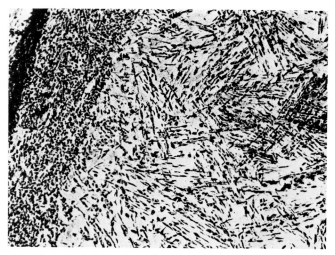

Figure 15-21. Flat (tangential) section of an experimental graft during rejection of the stroma. Vessels, fibroblasts, and round cells originating in the scar invade the stroma (Silver carbonate of Rio Hortega, ×100).

cells, and fibroblasts invaded the stroma in later stages of graft rejection (Fig. 15-21). Alterations of stromal fibers were also seen in late stages of rejection; lamellae were swollen due to edema and possibly due to proteolytic enzymes released during cell destruction.

Transmission electron microscopy of the superficial corneal graft stroma showed destruction of the epithelial basement membrane through which fibrocytes seem to migrate from rejecting stroma to rejecting basement epithelial cells. The area of stromal rejection showed a conglomeration of lymphocytes and altered corneal cells (Fig. 15-22). Lymphocytes showed cytoplasmic processes and were in intimate contact with keratocytes or with other lymphocytes. They

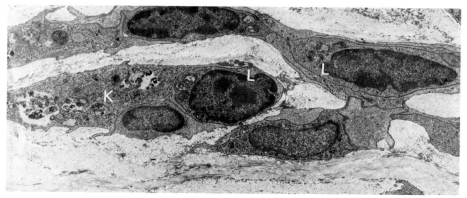

Figure 15-22. Lymphocytes (L) infiltrate the stroma of the graft. These cells attach to keratocytes (K), which show degenerative changes (TEM, ×6600). (Reproduced by permission.[42])

were round- or oval-shaped with a round or oval nucleus, condensed chromatin, several mitochondria granules, poorly developed Golgi complex, and scattered ribosomes. Severe cellular alterations were present in keratocytes in contact with lymphocytes; they showed distended endoplasmic reticulum, vacuoles, phagocytized material and high-density crystalline intracytoplasmic material. Typical plasma cells were not found in rejection areas; however, there were leukocytes that seemed to be intermediate forms of the lymphocytes and plasma cells. A discrete number of immunoblast-like cells were frequently found around the rejection area. They contained few ribosomes grouped in small clusters, scanty endoplasmic reticulum, and a few mitochondria.

The deeper stroma showed a moderate number of lymphocytes in contact with keratocytes or other lymphocytes. Disruption of the normal lamellar structure of the graft was evident in areas of leukocytic infiltration, even though edema was not evident. Altered keratocytes showed multiple cytoplasmic processes with rounding of the cell body, vacuolization, and phagocytized material.

New capillary vessels were found in the anterior and middle layers of stroma, where lymphocytes and plasma cells were seen predominantly outside the endothelial capillary wall. Some lymphocytes were present between the endothelial and the peri-endothelial vascular sheath and were surrounded by basement membrane. Typical plasma cells, some in mitotic stage, were seen around capillary walls or host stroma; in some other areas, there were clumps of immunoblast-like cells in areas of host stroma near vascular structures (see Fig. 15-8).

Ground Substance

The amount of ground substance or acid mucopolysaccharides present in host and grafted cornea was studied by the degree of metachromasia present in flat corneal sections stained with toluidine blue. Metachromatic staining of host and graft was even and similar in control corneas; however, grafts that were partially hazy showed a corresponding decrease or absence of metachromasia that became totally absent in opaque and rejected grafts.

The metachromatic reaction of toluidine blue indicates a quantity of mucopolysaccharides present in the cornea; however, it doesn't tell us the amount of sulfated substances being synthesized at a specific time. In a previous chapter, we have described the technique of radioactive sulfate (^{35}S) labeling of ground substance in order to study its turnover in the normal and in the grafted cornea. It was shown that most of this sulfate is incorporated in the keratan-18 sulfate or keratosulfate fraction of the ground substance. ^{35}S-labeled grafts, which became opaque as a result of an immune rejection, showed a decreased amount of radioactive sulfate incorporated in the hazy area still not invaded by fibrovascular tissue (Fig. 15-23**A–D**). However, transplants that became cloudy and eventually vascularized showed an increased uptake of sulfate, as it would be expected in a rapidly growing scar tissue. The radioactive sulfate used to label these animals had been injected intravenously (1 mCi/kg) at the beginning of the rejection process, after the graft had become completely opaque and vascularized, and in animals with clear grafts.

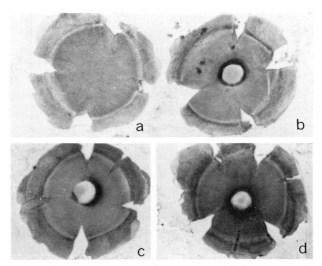

Figure 15-23. The ground substance of the cornea has been labeled with ^{35}S, and **A** shows the normal uptake of the isotope. **B.** A 4-wk-old corneal graft shows uptake similar to that of the host cornea. Scar tissue shows greater uptake. **C** and **D.** Decreased ^{35}S uptake by rejecting grafts. There is an increased uptake by scar tissue surrounding the graft.

Endothelium

The earliest change observed in the endothelial layer was a destruction of cells adjacent to the scar and at the periphery of the graft (Fig. 15-16). This was preceded by a line of leukocytic infiltration, predominantly of round cells that advanced towards the center of the graft (Fig. 15-24). This condition correlated well with the biomicroscopic observations that the haziness of the graft started near the scar. The white line seen in some grafts between two opaque areas or between the clear and the cloudy area, corresponded to a band or a line of leukocytes deposited on the endothelium (Figs. 15-25 and 15-26). In severe and rapid rejections, several polymorphonuclear leukocytes were often observed. Endothelial cells were of normal appearance in the clear area, but round cells were found scattered among them in the center of the graft. The cloudy portion of the graft showed an uneven posterior surface and cellular infiltration. Mononuclear leukocytes frequently infiltrated the endothelium, replacing cells in the more severely damaged portions in some areas of the opaque graft; Descemet's membrane was exposed to the anterior chamber. Endothelial cells were often rounded or globular. In other areas, there were clumps of lymphocytes, particularly in the junction between the normal and the cloudy area. As previously mentioned, it appeared that in a large number of rejecting grafts, the rejecting cells gained access to the endothelial surface through the host–graft junction. Whereas a well-healed, 4-wk-old endothelium covering the host-graft function shows none or a few white cells on its surface, the rejecting corneal graft shows swelling of this host–graft junction with prominent invasion of the scar

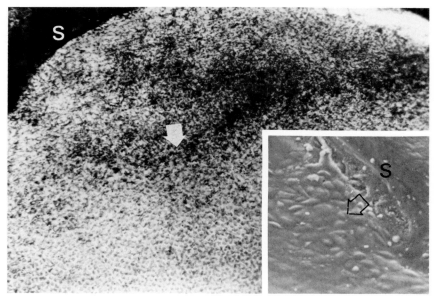

Figure 15-24. Flat endothelial preparation of a corneal graft at the beginning of the rejection. A line of white cells advances from the scar (S) towards the center of the graft (arrows). Insert shows round cells and fibroblasts advancing toward the center of the graft (hematoxylin and eosin, ×25; insert: SEM, ×200).

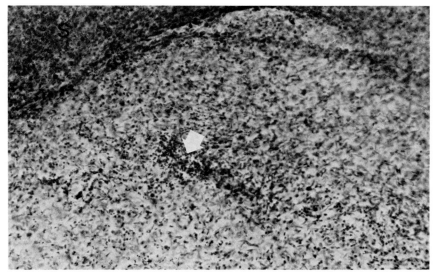

Figure 15-25. Flat endothelial preparation of an early graft rejection showing a clump of lymphocytes (arrow) near the scar. Line formation suggests that these cells arise from the wound area (hemotoxylin and eosin, ×100).

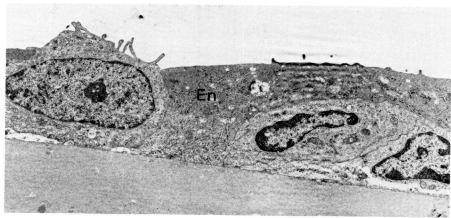

Figure 15-26. Lymphocytes between and under endothelial cells during the rejection process in an experimental graft. Endothelial cell (En) shows degenerative changes (TEM, ×2700).

and periphery of the graft with leukocytes. In the area of rejection, lymphocytes are present on the surface or between the endothelial cells. Often, they show part of the cytoplasm bulging into the anterior chamber and another portion touching Descemet's membrane (Figs 15-26 and 15-27). Endothelial cells in contact with lymphocytes show a cytoplasm of a higher density than that of normal endothelium and mitochondria with pale matrix and loss of cristae. Rejected endothelial cells appeared elongated or rounded with loss of their cell junctions

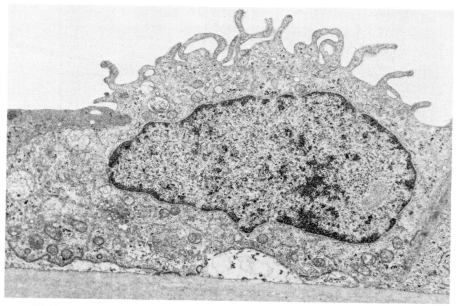

Figure 15-27. The cytoplasm of the lymphocytes bulges into the anterior chamber, while part of it remains attached to Descemet's membrane (TEM, ×4000).

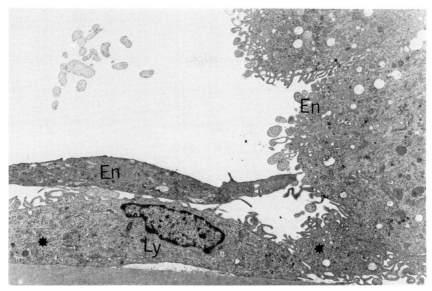

Figure 15-28. Area of active endothelial rejection (rejection line) showing destroyed endothelial cells (En) projected into the anterior chamber. Other cells in contact with lymphocytes (Ly) also show degenerative changes (*). (TEM, ×4750).

and many cytoplasmic processes (Fig. 15-28). Some of these cells with increased density appear free in the anterior chamber. They show mitochondria, endoplasmic reticulum, and vacuoles of different sizes. Lymphocytes of various shapes are also found free or between endothelial cells, but often they form a line between the rejected and the normal area (Fig. 15-29). This rejection line can be demonstrated in the scanning electron microphotograph of Figure 15-30. In Figures 15-31 and 15-32, endothelial cells are in the process of rejection.

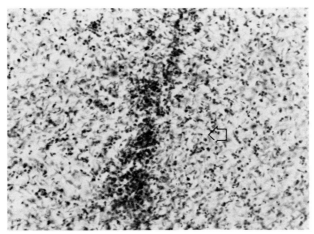

Figure 15-29. Typical rejection band or line in the endothelium as seen in a flat endothelial preparation stained with hematoxylin and eosin (×100).

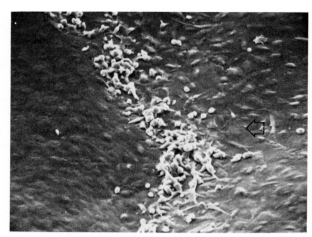

Figure 15-30. The same line as seen in Figure 15-29 under scanning electron microscopy. The arrow indicates the progression of the cells towards the normal area (SEM ×200).

Grafts with advanced rejection show abnormal endothelial cells over Descemet's membrane when examined by light microscopy. With the scanning electron microscope, Descemet's membrane appeared covered by abnormal endothelial cells and fibroblast-like elongated cells. With the transmission electron microscope, these cells do in fact appear to be fibroblasts; however, they have junctions typical of endothelial cells, cytoplasm of various densities, elongated nuclei, and a distended endoplasmic reticulum. They are often surrounded by collagen material and are frequently found in areas of retrocorneal fibrous membrane formation. Fully rejected grafts, when examined with the

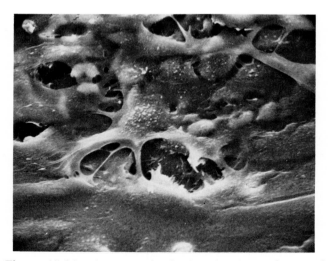

Figure 15-31. An area of rejection showing a destroyed endothelial cell surrounded by lymphocytes (SEM, ×500).

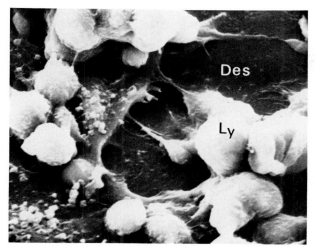

Figure 15-32. At higher magnification, a clump of lymphocytes (Ly) is shown over Descemet's membrane (Des) and around destroyed endothelial cells (SEM, ×2000).

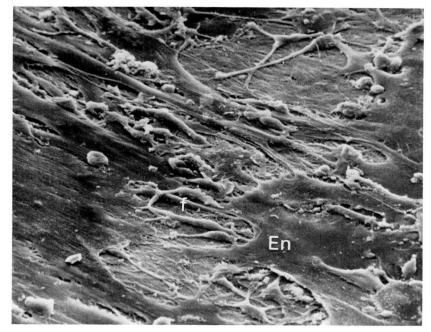

Figure 15-33. Endothelial surface of a regraft case in a patient with advanced graft rejection. It shows abnormal endothelial cells (En), fibroblasts (f), inflammatory cells, and collagen fibers over Descemet's membrane (SEM, ×1300).

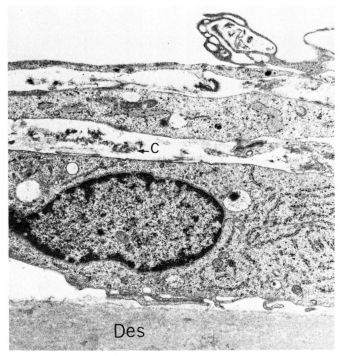

Figure 15-34.   Early retrocorneal fibrous membrane in a rejected human corneal graft. Cells with prominent endoplasmic reticulum are found over Descemet's membrane (Des) with interposed layers of collagen fibrils (c). (TEM, ×4200).

scanning electron microscope, show cells forming two or three layers among fibrous tissue between them (Fig. 15-33). This is confirmed with the transmission electron microscope, where one can see two or three layers of fibroblasts and endothelial cells with a thin fibrous layer between them and Descemet's membrane and over their surface exposed to the anterior chamber (Fig. 15-34). These fibroblasts have a distended endoplasmic reticulum, several mitochondria, a well developed Golgy complex, and filaments near the cell membrane. In other areas, Descemet's membrane appears covered by a thick fibrinous layer and regenerated endothelial cells.

DISCUSSION

Improvements in surgical techniques, suture material, and better selection of donor tissue have decreased the frequency of early graft failures. It is well accepted today that graft edema immediately following keratoplasty is the result of abnormal donor endothelium, complications during surgery, anterior segment inflammation, or faulty surgical technique. Once the graft is incorporated and remains clear for several weeks, there are few conditions that may cause its opacification, the most frequent cause being the immune reaction.[18,30] We estimate that in good prognosis cases, the frequency of graft rejections is around

12%,[11] a figure that is similar to that found by other authors.[9,18] The graft reaction is an immunologic process, as it has been demonstrated in our experiments and those of others.[1,8,17,20,23] Even though, clinically, there are no diagnostic tests of rejection, clinical signs (such as an inflammatory process and edema confined to the transplant, the edema of the graft that starts near the scar, and a typical rejection line frequently observed in the endothelium) are very useful clinical signs (almost pathognomic) to make a definite diagnosis, particularly if the transplant has previously been clear. In our experience, rejections have been more frequent after the fifth postoperative week; whereas, in other series, it occurred as early as 3 wk.[18] It is well known that the morbidity and characteristics of the immune graft reaction vary with the use of steroids and the anatomic condition of the recipient cornea, vascularization being one of the most important factors in the development of the immune reaction. According to Khodadoust,[18] the incidence of rejections in avascular corneas is 3.5%, whereas in mildly vascularized corneas, it was 13.3% and 65% in heavily vascularized corneas. The importance of corneal vascularization in the host has been emphasized by several authors.[1-6,8,9] The other factor that seems to account for a large number of graft rejections is a defective wound.[11,33] According to Kurz and D'Amico,[34] a defective host–graft alignment was found in 100% of failed grafts examined histopathologically. Even though the diagnosis of past graft reaction cannot be made in routine histologic sections of opaque grafts, their observations support our findings that in many instances of typical graft rejection, the rejection process started in the area of defective wound, iris synechiae, or previous wound rupture.[8] The elevated incidence of graft rejection in keratoconus (35%) reported by Chandler and Kaufman[35] and the 31% reported by Offret and Pouliquen,[33] can be explained by defective healing or a very large graft misalignment because most surgeons consider these values rather high. As previously mentioned, severely vascularized corneas will show a high incidence of rejection, which tends to increase in recipients with active inflammation, previous surgery, large grafts, and an abnormal host response to the transplantation procedure. In our experience, transplants done in recipients with poor prognosis will show rejections higher than 75%; however, it is difficult to be certain of the cause of graft opacification, because many of these transplants were not clear immediately after surgery.

Clinical and experimental studies indicate that the mechanism of rejection is mediated by lymphatic tissue that appears hyperplastic before the graft rejection. In our experimental set-up, it appears that vascularization of the host cornea is a prerequisite for the immune reaction, and in most clinical cases, this seems to be true. Our observations seem to support the theory that immunologic competent cells (small lymphocytes and plasma cells) must be in contact with the graft tissue in order to cause it destruction. Since lymphatic channels have been demonstrated in vascularized corneas, it is possible that these lymphatic cells, possibly originating in lymphoid centers around the cornea, may reach the graft through these channels and penetrate the anterior chamber through the scar with its unhealed Descemet's membrane. Grafts with abnormal healing or poor alignment of the posterior host–graft junction would be more susceptible to the migration of these cells to the graft endothelium. These have been shown experimentally by light and electron microscopy, and our experimental studies seem to support the concept that a properly aligned graft will have a better regeneration of Descemet's membrane, thus making the access of these cells to the anterior chamber more difficult.[11,32,33]

It is well known, however, that graft reactions in the human can also develop in avascular corneas,[2] but they have a different clinical appearance. Edema in these grafts may be associated to ciliary congestion and scattered KPs,[27] but occasionally, we may see a graft that developed diffuse edema without KPs. In these cases, we may suspect that endothelial damage has been caused by antibodies circulating in the anterior chamber. Tsutsui and Watanabe[36] found antibodies to grafted corneas in the serum of the host, and Smith and Woodin[37] showed that antibodies could be evoked by corneal extracts. In experimental grafts, we found that increased amounts of IgG was present in the aqueous humor of eyes with transplanted corneas at the time of rejection,[32] and recently, it has been shown that the aqueous humor of rabbit eyes undergoing graft rejection has the effect of inhibiting the migration of lymphocytes in vitro.[38] Anticorneal antibodies can damage endothelial cells under certain conditions, as described by Manski et al.[26] In their experiments, these antibodies could destroy the corneal endothelium in vivo only if these cells had been previously altered by trauma or were in the process of recovering from trauma or inflammation. It is possible, therefore, that high levels of circulating antibodies may affect abnormal corneal endothelium causing graft cloudiness.

The late stages of endothelial cell destruction by the inflammatory process are characterized by the presence of fibroblast-looking endothelial cells and the formation of retrocorneal membranes. In most instances, the rejection process can be reversed with steroids, and the graft can recover transparency; however, if the rejection process has advanced to the stage of posterior graft membrane formation with stromal infiltration and vascularization, opacification will be permanent. In some cases of severely vascularized corneas with profound structural alterations (chemical burns), irreversible opacification usually occurs despite proper immunosuppressive and steroid treatment.

Immunosuppression of the Graft Rejection

Graft rejection is a complex phenomenon; and antibody response is only one step in the process of graft destruction. Some types of antigens cause the release of host antibodies that will activate immune lysis by complement fixation, while others will aglutinate bacteria or cause anaphylactic sensitization.[46] Except for the reports of Tsutsui and Watanabe[38] and Smith and Woodin,[39] most investigators have not found circulating antibodies in corneal allografts. The lack of circulating antibodies may possibly occur because they are easily bound to the host's own cells or mask antibody molecules. It is accepted that graft destruction is mediated by competent T cells, and specific immunosuppression has been directed to their destruction (by steroids, x-rays, radiomimetic drugs) by inhibiting their proliferation (antimetabolites) or by their inactivation (antilymphocyte serum). At the present time, treatment is limited mostly to the use of steroids and, to a lesser extent, the use of immunosuppressive agents (Cytoxan, azathioprine, 6-mercapto-purine, and antilymphocyte serum).

Heterologous antilymphocytic serum has been used in other clinical fields in conjunction with immunosuppression.[47,48] Its clinical application is limited by its immunogenicity. We have used antilymphocytic serum experimentally with satisfactory results,[49] as have other investigators.[50-54] Its use in clinical corneal graft rejection has not been the subject of a detailed study.

Azathioprine (Imuran) is the antimetabolite most frequently used to modify the corneal immune reaction.[55-62] This drug has been used experimentally alone or in combination with steroids.[55] The topical or subconjunctival use of these antimetabolites has been ineffectual in preventing experimental graft rejections.[56,62] Elliot and Leibowitz[62] reported good results on the use of the antimetabolite in 12 cases that were considered unfavorable for penetrating keratoplasty because of the severity of scarring and vascularization of the recipient cornea. They used a priming dose of 6-10 mg/kg of body weight, with a daily dose of 0.5-4 mg/kg. The treatment was continued for 21 days to 4 mo. Urrets-Zavalia also used azathioprine in 16 cases of penetrating keratoplasty in unfavorable cases and reported that at least one of them was improved by the treatment. Other authors,[65-67] have also used the drug in a limited form; however, its use has not been widely accepted.

Steroids are the most valuable form of treatment of graft rejection when the diagnosis has been made early.[68] Even if steroids could reverse the immune reaction, the alterations would be irreversible in cases of advanced graft disease. Because the graft rejection compromises the lymphoid system of the entire body, systemic steroid treatment is frequently needed. In cases of mild rejection, however, the frequent administration of topical steroids can control the rejection process.

Corticosteroids suppress the graft reaction by their nonspecific antiinflammatory effect and by decreasing the level of serum complement. The hormone also interferes with the recognition of antigens on macrophage surfaces,[69] decreases the production of interferon, and most importantly, decreases the proliferation of lymphocytes by interfering with DNA synthesis and by its cytolytic effect on certain populations of small lymphocytes. Burton et al.[70] demonstrated that the destruction of T lymphocytes was a direct effect on the cell membrane, similar to the cell lysis caused with x-irradiation.[71-72] In a series of experiments,[73] we treated rejecting corneal grafts with the repeated instillation of topical 0.1% dexamethasone. This treatment improved the graft edema and decreased the number of endothelial infiltrates, thus supporting clinical observations that a similar application of topical steroids can reverse mild graft rejection in humans. When the endothelium of experimental grafts treated with steroids was examined with the scanning electron microscope, a decreased number of lymphocytes was revealed when compared with controls. There were lymphocytes in various stages of destruction (Fig. 15-35) and cell residues among regenerating endothelial cells. The lympholytic effect of topically applied steroids explains the rapid disappearance of inflammatory cells from the graft endothelium and corneal thinning during the immune reaction.[74] It is apparent that this type of steroid can penetrate the cornea, reach the anterior chamber, and destroy the effector lymphocytes; however, systemic steroids are frequently needed to block the release of such cells from the uveal tissue or from the vascularized host cornea. The most favorable cases for graft rejection suppression with corticosteroids are grafts in eyes with mild vascularization and/or with a trans-

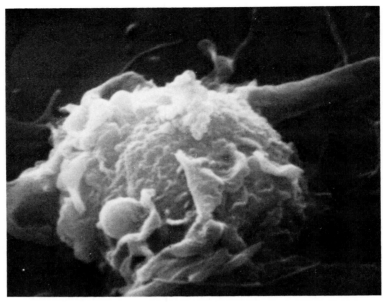

Figure 15-35. Lymphocyte in a corneal graft treated with topical steroids, showing cytoplasmic rupture and extrusion of nuclear chromatin (SEM, ×5000).

plant of less than 8 mm in size.[68] Graft recovery also depends on the number and quality of donor cells; repeated rejection episodes may destroy large numbers of endothelial cells, and, eventually, the graft will opacify.

Patients with corneal transplants are advised to immediately report any change in visual acuity, eye discomfort, light sensitivity, or eye redness. The appearance of these symptoms and signs is indicative of an immune reaction unless proven otherwise. A careful slit-lamp examination and pachymetry may reveal the findings previously described in this chapter. In this situation, we start the instillation of 0.1% dexamethasone sodium phosphate (Decadron) every hour during the daytime and 0.05% Decadron ointment at bedtime; in addition, we administer an intravenous injection of 40 mg of methylprednisolone sodium succinate, U.S.P. (Solu-Medrol), as recommended by Buxton et al.[75]

Silk sutures are often the inciting cause of this immune reaction, and they must be removed if the wound appears strong. Sometimes, this type of suture must be removed as early as 6–8 wk after keratoplasty, particularly in young persons or children. If graft edema and keratic precipitates have disappeared within 48 hr, the frequency of topical steroid administration is reduced, but it is continued for several weeks. Patients with keratoconus, vascularized corneas, repeated grafts, and some patients with corneal edema must continue the use of topical steroids (1 drop a day) for periods of 10–12 mo. Since the effect of steroids is mostly lympholytic and since they severely interfere with corneal healing, we do not pretreat eyes to be grafted (unless they are very vascularized), in contrast to Moore and Aronson's reports.[75]

If the immune reaction does not seem to improve with the topical application and the intravenous injection of Solu-Medrol alone, oral corticosteroids (prednisone) are started at levels of 60–80 mg/day in addition to the topical steroids. As soon as some improvement in the thickness of the graft is evident, the systemic steroids are decreased and tapered over a course of 2–3 wk, while maintaining the topical steroids. During this period of time, the intraocular pressure must be monitored. The possibility that the patient may have secondary bacterial infection should always be considered.

REFERENCES

1. Maumenee AE: The influence of donor–recipient sensitization on corneal grafts. Am J Ophthalmol 34:142, 1951
2. Maumenee AE: Clinical aspects of the corneal homograft reaction. Invest Ophthalmol 1:244, 1962
3. Castroviejo R: Atlas of Keratectomy and Keratoplasty. Philadelphia, Saunders, 1966, pp 404–405
4. DeVoe AG: *In* King JH, McTigue JW (eds): The Cornea World Congress. The Present Status of Keratoplasty. Washington, Butterworths, 1965, pp 332
5. Paton RT: Keratoplasty. New York, McGraw-Hill, 1955, p 231
6. Buxton JN, Chambers CF: *In* Bronson NR II, Paton RT (eds): Advances in Keratoplasty. Boston, Little, Brown, 1970, p 199
7. Offret G, Pouliquen Y, Guyot D: Aspects cliniques des reactions immunitaires apres keratoplasties transfixiantes chez l'homme. Arch Ophtalmol (Paris) 30:209, 1970
8. Polack FM: Histopathological and histochemical alterations in the early stages of corneal graft rejection. J Exp Med 116:709, 1962
9. Fine M, Stein M: The role of corneal vascularization in human corneal graft reactions. *In* Porter R, Knight J (eds): Corneal Graft Failure, Ciba Foundation Symposium. New York, Elsevier, Excerpta Medica, North-Holland, 1973, pp 151–163
10. Khodadoust AA: The allograft rejection reaction: The leading cause of late failure of clinical grafts. *In*: Porter R, Knight J (eds): Corneal Graft Failure, Ciba Foundation Symposium. New York, Elsevier, Excerpta Medica, North Holland, 1973, pp 151–163
11. Polack FM: Clinical and pathological aspects of the corneal graft reaction. Trans Am Acad Ophthalmol 77:418, 1973
12. Gowans JL, McGregor DD, Cowers DM: *In*: Wolstenholme G, Knight J (eds): The Immunologically Competent Cell: Its Nature and Origin. The role of small lymphocytes in the rejection of homografts of skin. London, Churchill, 1963, p 20
13. Medawar PB: *In* Wolstenholme G, Knight J (eds): Introduction. The Immunologically Competent Cell: Its Nature and Origin. London, Churchill, 1963
14. Gowans JL: The role of lymphocytes in the destruction of homografts. Br Med J 21:106, 1965
15. Polack FM, Gonzales CE: The response of the lymphoid tissue to corneal heterografts. Arch Ophthalmol 80:321, 1968
16. Paufique L, Sourdille P, Offret G: Les Greffes de la Corneé. Paris, Masson et Cie, 1948
17. Mueller M, Maumenee AE: Considerations sur le maladie de greffon. Arch Ophtalmol (Paris) 2:146, 1951
18. Khodadoust AA: Lamellar corneal transplantation in the rabbit. Am J Ophthalmol 66:1111, 1968
19. Polack FM: Inhibitions of immune corneal graft rejection by azathioprine. Arch Ophthalmol 74:683, 1965

20. Khodadoust AA, Silverstein AM: The survival and rejection of epithelium in experimental corneal transplants. Invest Ophthalmol 8:169, 1969

21. Casey TA: Discussion: Role of corneal vascularization, (Fine and Stein). *In* Porter R, Knight J (eds): Corneal Graft Failure. Ciba Foundation Symposium. New York, Elsevier, Excerpta Medica, North-Holland, 1973, p 207

22. Maumenee AE: Discussion: Role of corneal vascularization. *In* Porter R, Knight J (eds): Corneal Graft Failure. Ciba Foundation Symposium. New York, Elsevier, Excerpta Medica, North-Holland, 1973, p 208

23. Moore TE, Aronson SB: The corneal graft. A multiple variable analysis of the penetrating keratoplasty. Am J Ophthalmol 72:1, 1971

24. Medawar PB: Immunity to homologous grafted skin. III. The fate of skin homografts transplanted to the brain, to subcutaneous tissue, and to the anterior chamber of the eye. Br J Exp Pathol 29:50, 1948

25. Elliott JH, Flax MH, Leibowitz HM: The limbal cellular infiltrate in experimental cellular hypersensitivity. I. Morphological studies after primary immunization. Arch Ophthalmol 76: 104, 1966

26. Parks JL, Leibowitz HM, Maumenee AE et al: A transient stage of delayed hypersensitivity during the early induction of immediate corneal sensitivity. J Exp Med 115:867, 1962

27. Howes EL: Cellular hypersensitivity in the cornea. An analysis of the limbus and limbal cellular infiltration by light and electron microscopy. Arch Ophthalmol 83:475, 1970

28. Gowans JL, McGregor DD, Cowen DM, et al: Initiation of immune responses by small lymphocytes. Nature 196:654, 1962

29. Manski W, Ehrlich G, Polack FM: Studies on the cytotoxic immune reactions: I. The action of antibodies on normal and regenerating corneal tissue. J Immunol 105:755, 1972

30. Offret G, Pouliquen Y, Guyot D: Aspects cliniques des reactions immunitaires apreas keratoplasties transfixiantes chez l'homme. Arch Ophtalmol (Paris) 30:209, 1970

31. Khodadoust AM, Silverstein A: Induction of corneal graft rejection by passive cell transfer. Invest Ophthalmol 14:573, 1976

32. Polack FM, Smelser GK, Rose J: Long-term survival of isotopically-labelled stromal and endothelial cells in corneal homografts. Am J Ophthalmol 57:67, 1964

33. Hanna C: Fate of stromal cells in rabbit lamellar corneal grafts. Am J Ophthalmol 60:39, 1965

34. Graf B, Pouliquen Y, Frouin MA, et al: The phenomena of reabsorption in the course of cicatrization of experimental wounds of the cornea. Exp Eye Res 13:24, 1972

35. Offret G, Pouliquen Y: Les Homogreffes de la Corneé. Paris, Masson et Cie, 1974

36. Kurz GH, D'Amico R: Histopathology of corneal graft failures. Am J Ophthalmol 76:184, 1968

37. Chandler JW, Kaufman HE: Graft reactions after keratoplasty for keratoconus. Am J Ophthalmol 77:543, 1974

38. Tsutsui J, Watanabe S: Clinical evaluation of the precipitin test in the postoperative course of keratoplasty. Acta Soc Ophthalmol Jap 63:1950, 1959

39. Smith CR, Woodin AM: A note on th antigenic properties of corneal extracts. Br J Exp Pathol 34:647, 1953

40. Polack FM: Corneal graft rejection: Clinico-pathological correlation, *In* Porter R, Knight J (eds): Corneal Graft Failure. Ciba Foundation Symposium. New York, Elsevier, Excepta Medica, North-Holland, 1973, pp 127–139

41. Sher NA, Doughman D, Mindrup E, et al: Macrophage migration inhibition factor

activity in the aqueous humor during experimental corneal xenograft and allograft rejection. Am J Ophthalmol 82:858, 1976

42. Kanai A, Polack FM: Ultramicroscopic changes in the corneal graft stroma during early rejection. Invest Ophthalmol 10:415, 1971

43. Inomata H, Smelser GK, Polack FM: Corneal vascularization in experimental uveitis and graft rejection. Invest Ophthalmol 10:840, 1971

44. Inomata H, Smelser GK, Polack FM: Fine structure of regenerating endothelium and Descemet's embrane in normal and rejecting corneal grafts. Am J Ophthalmol 70:48, 1970

45. Kanai A, Polack FM: Ultramicroscopic alterations of corneal epithelium in corneal grafts. Am J Ophthalmol 72:119, 1971

46. Hager EB: *In* Hanna C (ed): Immunosuppression: Symposium of suppression of graft rejection. Baltimore, Williams & Wilkins, 1966, p 415

47. Starzl TE, Porter KA, Iwasaki Y, et al: The use of heterologous antilymphocytic globulin in human renal homotransplantation, *In* Wolstenholme GEW, O'Connor M (eds): Antilymphocytic Serum. Boston, Little, Brown, 1967

48. Kashiwagi N, Brantigan CO, Bieffsehneider L, et al: Clinical reactions and serologic changes after the administration of heterologous antilymphocyte globulin to human recipients of renal homografts. Ann Lut Med 68:275, 1968

49. Polack FM: Heterologous antilymphocyte serum, *In* Kaufman HE (ed): Ocular Anti-Inflammatory Therapy. Springfield, Ill, Charles C Thomas, 1970, p 130

50. Smolin G: Suppression of corneal graft reaction by antilymphocyte serum. Arch Ophthalmol 79:603, 1968

51. Smolin G: Suppression of the corneal homograft reaction by anti-lymphocytic serum. Ach Ophthalmol 81:571, 1969

52. Bell GC, Elliot JH: The effect of antilymphocytic serum on the corneal xenograft reaction. Invest Ophthalmol 7:112, 1968

53. Vannas S, Merenmies L, Tilikainen A, et al: The effect of homologous anti-lymphocytic serum on rabbit corneal heterografts. Acta Ophthalmol 47:93, 1969

54. Waltman S, Faulkner HW, Burde RM: Modification of the ocular immune response I. Use of antilymphocytic serum to prevent immune rejection of penetrating homografts. Invest. Ophthalmol 8:196, 1969

55. Polack FM: Effect of azathioprine (Imuran) on corneal graft reaction. Am J Ophthalmol 64:233, 1967

56. Polack FM: Inhibition of immune corneal graft rejection by azathioprine (Imuran). Arch Ophthalmol 74:683, 1965

57. Cleasby GW, Byland SS: Corneal transplantation in modified recipients. Invest Ophthalmol 3:460, 1964 (abstract)

58. D'Amico RA, Castroviejo R: Suppression of the immune response in keratoplasty. Am J Ophthalmol 68:829, 1969

59. Elliot JH: Immunosuppressive therapy of ocular inflammatory diseases: An alternative? Arch Ophthalmol 81:612, 1969

60. Leibowitz HM, Elliott JH: Antimetabolite suppression of corneal hypersensitivity. Arch Ophthalmol 73:94, 1965

61. Elliot JH, Leibowitz HM, Boruchoff SA, et al: Penetrating keratoplasty with adjunctive azathioprine (Imuran) therapy—a preliminary report. *In* Kaufman HE (ed): Ocular Anti-inflammatory Therapy. Springfield, Ill, Charles C Thomas, 1970 pp 169–191

62. Elliot JH, Leibowitz HM: Immunosuppression of corneal graft rejection: Clinical and experimental. *In* Dabezies OH, Gitter KA, Samson CLM (eds): Symposium on the Cornea. Transactions of the New Orleans Academy of Ophthalmology. St. Louis, C. V. Mosby, 1972, p 53

63. Urrets-Zavalia A Jr: Panel-nine, *In* King JH, McTigue JW (eds): The Cornea World Congress. Washington, Butterworth, 1965

64. MacKay IR, Bignell JL, Smith PH, et al: Prevention of corneal graft failure with the immunosuppressive drug azathioprine. Lancet 2:479, 1967

65. Hughes WF, Kallmeyer J: Etiology and treatment of the corneal homograft reaction including azathioprine (Imuran). South Afr Med J 41:548, 1967

66. Barraquer J: Personal communication, 1976

67. Gastaldi GM: L'impiego del trattamento immunodepressivo con azathioprina in alcuni casi di reazione infiamatorie dopo cheratoplastica perforate. Minerva Oftal 6:223, 1969

68. Maumenee AE: The role of steroids in the prevention of corneal graft failure, *In* Porter R, Knight J (eds): Corneal Graft Failure, Ciba Foundation Symposium. New York, Elsevier, Excerpta Medica, North-Holland, 1973, pp 241–255

69. Berenbaum MC: The biological basis of immunosuppression, *In* Porter R, Knight J (eds): Corneal Graft Failure. Ciba Foundation Symposium. New York, Elsevier, Excerpta Medica, North-Holland, 1973, pp 257–277

70. Burton AF, Storr JM, Dunn WL: Cytolytic actions of corticosteroids on thymus and lymphoid cells in vitro. Can J Biochem 45:289, 1967

71. Whitfield JF, Perris AD, Youdale DT: Destruction of the nuclear morphology of thymic lymphocytes by the corticosteroid cortisol. Exp Cell Res 52:349, 1968

72. Whitfield JF, Youdale DT, Perris AD: Early post-irradiation changes leading to the loss of nuclear structure in rat thymocytes. Exp Cell Res 48:461, 1967

73. Polack FM: Lymphocyte destruction during corneal homograft reaction: A scanning electron microscopic study. Arch Ophthalmol 89:413–416, 1973

74. Wind CA, Wood TO: Effects of steroids on corneal thickness following penetrating keratoplasty. Invest Ophthalmol 10:157, 1971

75. Buxton JN, Apisson JH, Hoeffle FB: Corticosteroids in 100 keratoplasties. Am J Ophthalmol 67:46, 1969

76. Moore TE, Aronson SB: Steroid therapy in penetrating keratoplasty. Trans Pac Coast Oto Opthalmol Soc 49:289, 1968

PART 4

Organization and Operation of an Eye Bank

Chapter 16

Preservation of Corneal Tissue

STORAGE OF EYES AT 4°C

When eyes are received in the eye bank, the technician takes a culture of the corneal surface, records the data in a log book, and evaluates the eye with the slit lamp and the specular microscope before they are treated with a topical antibiotic (Neosporin®, polymyxin B, neomycin, gramicidin). The eyes are then stored in a special jar (moist chamber) where the eye can be supported by a metal holder (Fig. 16-1) with the cornea facing up. The flexible aluminum holder has two small bars that must be gently bent in to hold the globe. In this model, the holder has a hole in its base through which the optic nerve is passed and secured with a small pin. A small amount of saline solution is placed in the bottom of the jar to produce some moisture.

If the eyes are referred to a distant hospital or eye bank, the tissue must be packed with ice in a styrofoam box, which is the most commonly used container in the United States (Fig. 16-2). Most of the eyes submitted for penetrating keratoplasty in this way are used within 24 hr; few are used between 24 and 48 hr. We can roughly estimate that 75% of eye bank eyes are used for penetrating keratoplasties, while the remaining ones are used for lamellar grafts, research, or are unsuitable for keratoplasty. If the eyes have not been treated with antibiotics before delivery to the surgeon, he should be notified so appropriate antibiotic treatment is given to the eye before surgery.

The topical application of a broad spectrum antibiotic (Neosporin) is now the preferred method of treatment instead of that of immersing the eye in an antiseptic solution. As the number of transplants being done with corneas excised in the laboratory increases, the treatment of donor eyes in the operating room will eventually decrease, and we will depend more and more on the proper sterility of the donor cornea. I like to consider the globe contaminated in spite of antibiotic treatment of the cornea at the eye bank. Intact globes are still sent to the operating room, and the surgeon should do his best to assure sterility of the donor cornea. In the operating room, the globe is wrapped in a long piece of gauze exposing only the cornea, then, with another sterile gauze, the superficial epithelium is removed, and frequent instillations of Neosporin solution are applied before the cornea is either excised for an endothelial graft cut (Fig. 8-1) or the graft is cut from the anterior surface with a trephine (Fig. 11-4**A–D**).

MEDIUM-TERM CORNEAL STORAGE

Some of the earlier reports on the preservation of excised corneas in a liquid medium go back to 1911, when Magitot[1] described a method of storing corneas in hemolyzed blood at 5°–8°C. Stallard[2] preserved isolated corneas in liquid paraffin

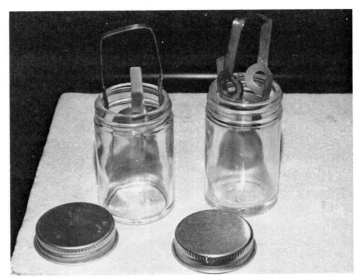

Figure 16-1. Moist chamber jars for eye storage at 4°C.

at 4°C. In Japan in 1961, Kuwahara[3] stored animal corneas in donor serum for several days with the purpose of decreasing the antigenicity of the donor tissue. This idea was utilized by Stocker, who in 1965,[4] incubated donor corneas in the prospective recipient's serum, not only to decrease the antigenicity of the tissue, but also to extend the storage time. According to Stocker, corneas kept in serum at 4°C would keep normal viability for as long as 1 wk. In 1963, I kept several rabbit corneas in rabbit serum for periods of 2–3 wk, following which penetrating keratoplasties were performed. Even though the transplants were slightly

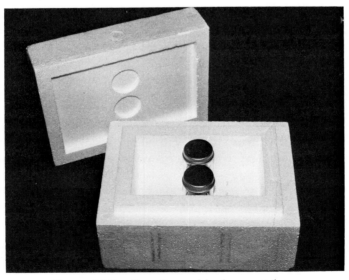

Figure 16-2. Styrofoam shipping container.

hazy on the first few days after keratoplasty, they all remained clear. It is known, however, that rabbit corneas with few endothelial cells can still give clear grafts. The most important item in this storage technique is sterility; Stocker[4] recommended the decontamination of the eye with a broad spectrum antibiotic solution before putting the excised cornea in the recipient serum. The container was then closed and placed in the refrigerator at 4°C. In 1965, Robbins et al.,[5] using NBT staining, evaluated the endothelium of rabbit corneas stored in serum for periods of 2–3 wk and found that for this long period of time, there was almost no difference in the survival of cells when compared to the whole rabbit eye kept in moist chamber for a similar period of time. Kobayashi[6] also evaluated this method of storage of rabbit corneas in 1964 and found that electron microscopic changes were acceptable up to 72 hr of serum storage time; but for longer periods of time, the alterations were too pronounced. In 1974, Van Horn and Schultz[7] compared cat corneas kept in moist chambers versus cat corneas stored in cat serum for different periods of time and concluded that the serum storage method did not afford any advantage over the moist chamber storage, at least during the period of time within 160 hr.

Kuwahara et al.,[8] in 1965, followed their studies of corneal incubation in serum with corneas incubated in artificial solutions for extension of cornea viability. Their solution was a basic tissue culture medium with a concentration of mucopolysaccharides similar to that found in corneal stroma, possibly in order to control stromal swelling. They reported their results on human penetrating keratoplasties after storage time of 7 days, and their success rate in 50 patients was better than 78%.[8]

In 1974, Sakimoto et al.[9] and McCarey and Kaufman[10] reported two techniques of corneal storage for penetrating keratoplasty. Sakimoto's technique requires a special corneal holder and the use of a balanced salt solution with the addition of 5% Dextran. The special container would allow the solution to bathe only the epithelial side while the endothelial side of the corneas was in a moist chamber environment. The preservation technique described by McCarey and Kaufman[10] required the use of the tissue culture Medium 199 and the addition of 5% Dextran (Fig. 16-3). A broad spectrum antibiotic solution is added to this tissue culture medium at the time the cornea is stored. The tissue culture medium contains a certain amount of CO_2 to adjust the pH to 7.4; therefore, it is important that the fluid level in the container should be high enough to allow a very small amount of air between the fluid and the cap. Containers of the tissue culture medium can be stored in the refrigerator for several months. The corneas stored in the M-K medium can be used up to 1 wk. Most surgeons, however, are using these corneas within a maximum storage time of 4 days.

Results with the short-term preservation medium (M-K medium) have been extremely successful, and at the present time, this technique has been adopted by most of the eye banks in the United States. It has allowed patients to be scheduled for penetrating keratoplasties and tissue to be transported at long distances in refrigerated containers without worries about time to limit the usefulness of the donor tissue. The expenses of processing the tissue and handling the ever increasing requests for donor corneas have now introduced the charge of a fee for processing these eyes, a fee that is paid by the patient just as any other medicines or materials used during the operation.

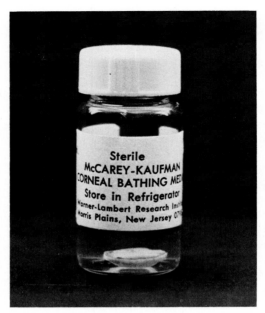

Figure 16-3. Container for corneal storage in tissue culture solution (M-K medium).

Preparation of the M-K Medium

1. Tissue culture Medium 199 (Microbiological Associates, Inc., Bethesda, Md.), 2× concentration without pH indicator.
2. Dextran 40, 5% (Sigma Chemical Company, St. Louis, Mo.).
3. Gentamicin, .1 mg/ml of medium.

Mix a 10% dilution of Dextran with equal parts of TC-199 (2× concentration). The final concentration is a 5% Dextran in TC-199 of normal concentration. The solution is sterilized through a Millipore filter (0.2 μ). The corneal storage vials will contain 20 cc of the M-K medium, and just before the cornea is immersed, 10,000 U (0.1 cc) of a streptomycin-penicillin mixture is added, (100 U/cc of medium) or Gentamycin, (.1 mg/ml of medium).

Another medium-term preservation techniques was that of Burki[11] who, in 1947, recommended the use of paraffin oil, which remained liquid. The isolated cornea was kept at 4°C until the time of surgery, for periods of time that extended up to 60–72 hr. Rycroft,[12] Gormaz and Eggers,[13] and Stallard[14] reported the use of these corneas up to 3 wk. The risk of contamination, because this oil could not be sterilized and could cause irritation, has been the reason this technique was not popularized.

Organ-Cultured Corneas

Doughman et al.[15] reported initial satisfactory results of penetrating keratoplasties using corneas cultured at 37°C for several days. This incubation conserves the viability of the endothelium, stroma, and epithelium, but it causes a pronounced degree of swelling. Swelling disappears shortly after grafting or after immersion in M-K medium (with Dextran) for several minutes. The two main problems with this technique are the higher risk of tissue infection and handling a thick graft. No proof of decreased antigenicity has been presented so far.

LONG-TERM PRESERVATION OF VIABLE TISSUE: CRYOPRESERVATION

The main problem in preserving corneas or any other tissue at very low temperatures was the formation of ice inside and around the cell. In 1949, Polge et al.[16] showed that cock and bull spermatozoa could be preserved at dry ice temperatures ($-79°C$) if the cells were previously bathed in 10%–15% glycerol. They later reported that these cells were alive after 6 yr of storage at low temperatures. These findings, as well as the explanation of causes of damage to living cells during the slow cooling to low temperatures,[17] were applied to the preservation of red blood cells, a procedure that revolutionized handling and storage of human blood. While this basic investigation was progressing, Eastcott et al.,[18] Rycroft,[19] and Iliff et al.[20] obtained a few clear human lamellar and penetrating keratoplasties with corneas preserved at low temperatures in the presence of glycerol. Even though Stocker et al.[21] could culture some cells from glycerol-treated frozen corneas, he concluded that the tissue was good only for lamellar keratoplasty, due to the low survival rate of endothelial cells. Smelser and Ozanics (1957, personal communication) also concluded that these glycerol-treated frozen corneas were suitable only for lamellar keratoplasty. In 1959, Lovelock[22] found that an industrial solvent called dimethylsufoxide (DMSO) could be used for the protection of cells during the freezing at low temperatures. Smith et al.[23] studied the use of this cryophylactic agent for the preservation of corneas at low temperatures in 1963 and found good endothelial survival after the cornea had been stored at $-79°C$. Using this technique, successful experimental corneal grafts were performed by Mueller and Smith[24,25] in 1963 and 1964. Kaufman,[26] in 1966, and Mueller,[27] in 1967, reported successful corneal grafts in humans using the cryopreservation techniques with dimethylsufoxide. The solutions used for corneal preservation were basically the same, with different approaches to the techniques of preservation. Where Kaufman and associates excised the cornea to be run through solutions of increasing concentrations of dimethylsufoxide, the technique of Mueller and Smith required the solution to be perfused through the anterior chamber of the eye, which was preserved as a whole in dry ice. The excised corneas of the Kaufman et al. technique were stored in liquid nitrogen.

The cryopreservation method has been used at the University of Florida for several years with satisfactory results. However, the requirements for successful survival of a cornea through the cryopreservation technique required that the mate cornea should be studied to eliminate the possibility of endothelial disease. Corneas that were removed over 10 hr after death did not do well after preservation, and corneas from patients over 60 yr of age also did poorly after cryopreservation and thawing. In essence, only young and fresh material did well with this preservation technique. For the corneal endothelium to adequately survive the cryopreservation method, it was important to freeze the corneas, which had been soaked in solutions of increasing concentrations of DMSO-albumin-dextrose, at a rate not to exceed 5°/min. A lower cell survival was observed when the corneas were frozen at a faster or slower rate. The slower rate seemed to be better suited for the preservation of stromal cells.[28] The cryo-preserved corneas were left in the last of the four DMSO bathing solutions, and then submerged in liquid nitrogen. At the time of thawing, the glass vial was taken to the operating room in liquid nitrogen, and the serum and cornea thawed in a water bath of about 60°C, so the thawing could be effected in less than 1 min by constant agitation. The albumin containing DMSO was poured out of this glass vial, and normal human albumin was put into the vial to remove traces of DMSO. The cornea was then ready to be used in keratoplasty.

In order to ship liquid-nitrogen-preserved corneas, it was necessary to place them in special liquid-nitrogen-insulated containers and recommend a very strict thawing procedure.

Several instruments can be used for corneal cryopreservation as long as the rate of freezing can be controlled. We have used the Linde freezer, the Capella® freezer (Fig. 16-4), a Revco electric freezer; and Paton and Martinez[29] have used the Bailey automatic freezer.

The McCarey et al.[35] 1975 survey indicated that 94% of the eye banks use moist chamber stored eyes, and 71% are now using M-K-media-preserved eyes. Many eye banks use both systems, which accounts for the two high percentages. Less than 7% of all eye banks use cryopreservation, as this system has been almost completely replaced by the short-term preservation.

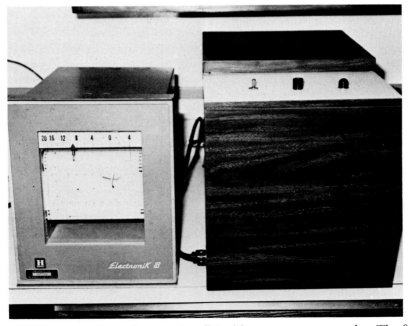

Figure 16-4. Controlled rate freezer (Capella) with temperature recorder. The freezing rate (5°/min) is monitored with a thermocouple.

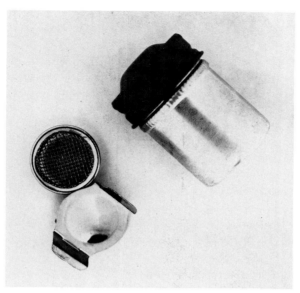

Figure 16-5.   Aluminum container and stainless steel wire basket for corneal storage and shipping in dry ice.

Modified Corneal Cryopreservation (Wire Basket Method)

The standard corneal cryopreservation method as used at the University of Florida[1] requires a trained technician to thaw the corneas properly, i.e., correct water temperature, avoid excessive tissue agitation, and avoid over warming the solution with DMSO. Transportation or mailing of these corneas should be done in special liquid-nitrogen-insulated containers. To avoid these difficulties, which may arise if no technician is available, or to simplify transportation, the cryopreservation method can be modified as follows:[36]

1. Pretreatment of corneas in each of the four preservative solutions with DMSO is done for 10 min at +4°C.
2. The cornea is removed from solution No. 4 (7.5% DMSO), and excess of fluid is quickly released from the tissue by touching the edge of sclera with a gauze.
3. It is then placed in a stainless steel wire basket (used for histologic processing of tissues)* and placed in a small aluminum container (photographic film container, Fig. 16-5), precooled at 4°C.
4. The metallic container is tightly closed and placed in the CR Freezer. The standard freezing curve is applied with the same reference electrode (Fig. 16-4).
5. At the end of the freezing procedure, the container is stored in liquid nitrogen.

*Micro-tissue capsules, Lipshaw Mfg. Co., Detroit, Cat. No. 331 (20 mm).

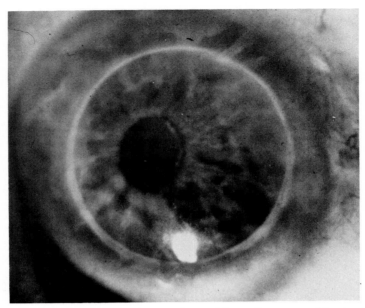

Figure 16-6.   Penetrating keratoplasty with graft preserved in dry ice.

From here, two steps can be followed: (1) use after thawing directly from liquid-nitrogen container, or (2) transfer to styrofoam container packed with dry ice for short-time storage, transport, or mailing.

The direct thawing from liquid nitrogen has given very good results experimentally, histologically, and clinically (Fig. 16-6). The possibilities of short-term dry-ice storage or shipping have been investigated and proven to be as satisfactory as liquid-nitrogen storage. Figure 16-7 **A–C** shows the steps in thawing, which essentially consist of placing the wire basket with the cornea in the patient's serum or in 25% human albumin at room temperature. This procedure thaws the cornea in 10 sec, partially hydrates the tissue, and releases the residual DMSO. The cornea then is ready for trephination and grafting.

REFERENCES

1. Magitot A: Sur la survie possible de la corneé transparente de l'oeil apres conservation prolongee en dehors de l'organisme. Soc Biol 70:46–48, 1911
2. Stallard HB: Eye Surgery. Baltimore, Williams & Wilkins, 1958, pp 400–401
3. Kuwahara Y: Studies of heterokeratoplasty. Jap J Ophthalmol 5:243, 1961
4. Stocker FW: Preservation of donor cornea in autologous serum prior to penetrating grafts. Am J Ophthalmol 60:21, 1965
5. Robbins JE, Capella JA, Kaufman HE: A study of endothelium in keratoplasty and corneal preservation. Arch Ophthalmol 73:242, 1965
6. Kobayashi S: Electron microscopy of stored corneal grafts. Acta Soc Ophthalmol Jap 68:952–964, 1964
7. Van Horn DL, Schultz RO: Comparison of serum versus eye bank storage of cat corneas. Arch Ophthalmol 92:114, 1974

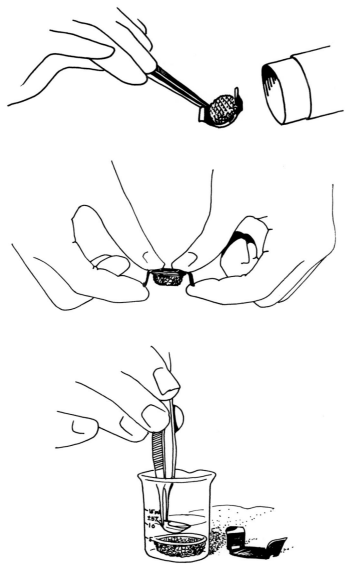

Figure 16-7. Thawing procedure of cyopreserved cornea stored in dry ice in aluminum container.

8.   Kuwahara Y, Sakanaue M: Studies on the long term preservation of the cornea for penetrating keratoplasty. Acta Soc Ophthalmol Jap 69:1751, 1965
9.   Sakimoto T, Valenti J, Itoi M, et al: Intermediate-term corneal storage. Invest Ophthalmol 13:219, 1974
10. McCarey BE, Meyer RF, Kaufman HE: Improved corneal storage for penetrating keratoplasties in humans. Ann Ophthalmol 8:1488–1495, 1976
11. Burki E: A new method of preserving corneal tissue. Ophthalmologica 114:288–293, 1947

12. Rycroft BW: The scope of corneal grafting. Br J Ophthalmol 38:1–9, 1954
13. Gormaz A, Eggers C: Eye bank. Arch Chil Oftal 16:47–53, 1959
14. Stallard HB: Eye Surgery. Baltimore, Williams & Wilkins, 1958, pp 414–415
15. Doughman DJ, Tani PM, Mindrup E: Immunologic modification of organ cultured rabbit cornea allografts. Presented at the Association for Research in Vision and Ophthalmology, April 26, 1974
16. Polge L, Lovelock JE: Preservation of bull sperm at −79 degrees centigrade. Vet Rec 64:396, 1952
17a. Lovelock JE: The haemolysis of human red blood-cells by freezing and thawing. Biochem Biophys Acta 10:414–426, 1953
17b. Lovelock JE: HET mechanism of the protective action of glycerol against haemolysis by freezing and thawing. Biochem Biophys Acta 11:28–36, 1953.
18. Eastcott HG, Cross AG, Leigh AG, et al: Preservation of corneal grafts by freezing. Lancet 1:237, 1954
19. Rycroft BW: Three unusual corneal grafts. J Ophthalmol 41:749, 1957
20. Iliff CE, Wood RM, Hollender DH: Successful transplantation of a frozen human cornea. Am J Ophthalmol 41:505, 1956
21. Stocker FW, King EH, Lucas DO, et al: Comparison of two different staining methods for evaluating corneal endothelial viability. Arch Ophthalmol 76:833, 1966
22. Lovelock JE, Bishop MWH: Prevention of freezing damage to living cells by dimethyl sulphoxide. Nature (Lond) 183:1394–1395, 1959
23. Smith AU, Ashwood-Smith MJ, Young MR: Some in vitro studies on rabbit corneal tissue. Exp Eye Res 2:71–87, 1963
24. Mueller FO, Smith AU: Some experimentation on grafting frozen corneal tissue in rabbits. Exp Eye Res 2:237, 1963
25. Mueller FO: Techniques for full thickness keratoplasty in rabbits using fresh and frozen corneal tissue. Br J Ophthalmol 48:377, 1964
26. Kaufman HE, Escapini H, Capella JA, et al: Living preserved corneal tissue for penetrating keratoplasty. Arch Ophthalmol 76:471, 1966
27. O'Neil P, Mueller FO, Trevor-Roper PD: On the preservation of cornea at −196 degrees centigrade for full thickness homografts in man and dog. Br J Ophthalmol 51:13, 1967
28. Polack FM, McEntyre JM: Incorporation of sodium sulfate S-35 by cryopreserved corneal grafts in vivo. Arch Ophthalmol 81:577–582, 1969
29. Paton RT, Martinez M: Corneal tissue preservation for penetrating keratoplasty, In Bellows JG (ed): Cryosurgery. 49:428–435, 1968
30. Amsler M, Verrey F: Le prelevement du greffon keratoplastique. Arch Ophtalmol (Paris) 8:150–151, 1948
31. Vannas M: Remarks on the technique of corneal transplantation. Am J Ophthalmol 33:70–71, 1950
32. Stallard HB: Eye Surgery. Baltimore, Williams & Wilkins, 1958, pp 405–406
33. Kaufman HE, Capella JA: Preserved corneal tissue for transplantation. J Cryosurg 1:125–129, 1968
34. Polack FM, Brightbill FM, Slappey T: A comparison of two methods for cutting donor corneal buttons. Am J Ophthalmol 75:3, 1973
35. McCarey BE, Marshall T: Eye bank survey 1974. Presented at the 1974 American Association of Eye Banks meeting, Dallas, Texas
36. Polack FM: Modified cryopreservation method, In Polack FM (ed): Corneal and External Diseases. Springfield, Ill, Charles C Thomas, 1969, pp 363–368

Chapter 17

Eye Bank Organization and Function

Eye Banks are nonprofit organizations whose two primary functions are to obtain human donor eyes and to make donor tissue available to qualified eye surgeons for transplantation purposes. Many eye banks are also centers for research on tissue preservation and eye pathology investigation, as well as places for training eye surgeons and eye bank technicians.

The Eye Bank for Sight Restoration, Inc. was organized in New York in 1945 by D. T. Paton and has served as a model for all the eye banks in the United States, which are grouped under the Eye Bank Association of America. Eye banks are usually organized as a response to needs for corneal tissue in certain communities; however, they could not exist if local laws did not encourage the removal of eye tissue. This has been the major drawback in organizing eye banks in other parts of the world, in addition to religious and social prejudices. Canada and most European countries have active eye banks with liberal laws to facilitate the removal of eye tissue. Since 1947, France has had legislation allowing the removal of eyes without next-of-kin permission if the patient died in a public institution and the body was not claimed within 24 hr. This waiting period could be modified by the director of the institution. An eye bank was organized in Australia in 1948, and in recent years, they have been organized in most Central and South American countries. In these countries, as well as in India[1] and the Middle East, although legislation authorized the removal of eyes, the need for next-of-kin consent and sociogeographic conditions usually delay the removal to a time past the usefulness of the cornea. These problems are now being smoothed out by the new eye banks through active educational campaigns.

In most countries, legislation to facilitate the procurement of human tissue for transplantation has been obtained through a long process of appeals, delays, and conflicts because of the nature of archaic laws and poor understanding of medical advances by the public and legislators. This problem is not unique to developing countries, but also exists in countries with advanced technology. Such was the case in the United States when heart transplantation became a reality. Laws were not clear as to the rights of an individual to donate organs at death, and ethical as well as moral issues confronted the surgeon. This issue may not apply to corneal transplantation, but as mentioned above, it is important to obtain legislation regulating autopsies, unclaimed bodies, and medical examiner cases. In 1968, the United States passed the Uniform Anatomical Gift Act in response to these shortcomings and the need for more human tissue.[2] This act supports the right of an individual to be able to control the disposition of all or part of his body upon his death. The act also gives the next-of-kin the authority to donate part or the whole body of the deceased, provided that the deceased had not expressed his desire against this donation. The mechanisms have also been regulated encouraging the process of tissue removal. In some countries, specific legislation to facilitate the removal of one organ, without permission of donor or next-of-kin, has been produced, as was the case in the Soviet Union. In 1937, they legalized the removal of eyes, as did several other countries where the legalization of eye removal was secured because there was a need to establish an eye bank.

ORGANIZATION

Persons interested in organizing an eye bank should draft bylaws to define the function of its directors, officers, and members (see appendix). The Board of Directors is composed of a President, Vice-President, and Secretary-Treasurer who are elected annually. On this Board, it is convenient to have an equal number of physicians and members of the community or from the service club that helps to organize the eye bank. In the United States, Lions International is the national service organization frequently associated with eye banks and sight preservation. The Board of Directors may appoint a Council Advisory Group (from the community) and a Committee of Sponsors, who are a group of citizens interested in helping and supporting the eye bank.

The function of the Medical Advisory Council is to deal with all medical and professional matters. The Medical Director is the officer of this Council, and he should be consulted on all matters pertaining to public relations and press releases for technical accuracy. The Executive Director is usually a full-time person in charge of all daily eye bank activities, who may also act as a technician if the size of the eye bank does not require additional personnel. The function of the Executive Director also includes a good working knowledge of public relations, the ability to give lectures on behalf of the eye bank at such civic organizations as the Rotary Clubs, Lions Clubs, Women's Clubs, etc.

ADMINISTRATION

The finances of the eye bank are controlled by the President and the Treasurer, but the Medical Director and other directors may have the power to sign checks if necessary. A bank account is opened in the name of the local eye bank and withdrawals and deposits are made only by authorized persons. The Internal Revenue Service office is contacted to secure tax-exempt status.

The administration of the eye bank is in the hands of the Medical Director, the Executive Director, and a technician. Usually, the eye bank is located in a medical center or in a hospital where a laboratory may be set up for eye examination and processing, the latter being the responsibility of the technician.

Once a central eye bank office is organized, the Board of Directors may want to request that local hospitals become affiliated with the eye bank to act as procurement stations. If necessary, branch eye banks can be set up; however, we have found at the University of Florida that a large number of eyes can be obtained through funeral directors (morticians) who have been trained and certified by the eye bank to remove eyes.

The Funeral Directors Program for eye enucleation was initiated in Iowa by Dr. Alson Braley, and at the present time, several medical centers (including ours) have a similar training program. Certified funeral directors are provided with enucleation instruments and shipping containers, which are returned to them after they deliver a set of eyes.

Eye banks are self-supporting institutions and require an operating capital, which is obtained through contributions, grants, or donations. A certain amount of advertising is required for the purpose of acquiring funds as well as to invite the community to complete pledges of eye donation. These activities must be under the auspices of the sponsoring civic organization and not directly by the ophthalmologists participating as medical directors. A well programmed public relations campaign can be effective in both areas using television and radio and by circulating pamphlets in the community.

SOURCE OF DONOR EYES

Most eye banks will obtain eyes from unrestricted postmortem autopsy permit by consent of relatives. In some areas, special permission must be obtained specifically for eye removal, in addition to the postmortem permit. Another common source is from persons whose eyes have been donated after death by the consent of relatives, whether or not an autopsy is required or requested. Other sources are persons who have bequeathed their eyes in writing before death under the Uniform Anatomical Gift Act and from medical examiner cases.

In the United States, some states allow the medical examiner's office to remove either the eye or the cornea for eye banks under certain conditions. Maryland was the first state to pass specific legislation establishing the authority of the medical examiner to remove corneal tissue when an autopsy is required to determine the cause of death. Texas and Florida now have similar legislation. The tantamount advancement to eye banking in this law is that the tissue may be taken without permission of next-of-kin.

Eye tissue made available from the medical examiners' offices will be the most important source of donor tissue in the near future. Autopsy cases handled through coroners' offices involve unattended deaths, deaths caused by accidents or violence. Since these cases often involve younger people in good health at the time of death, the tissue obtained from coroners' autopsies would, in many cases, more closely approximate the definition of "ideal" donor tissue.

EYE COLLECTION

An around-the-clock telephone answering service helps coordinate the donor's locations and the nearest physician or technician available to perform the eye removal. During working hours, all calls are taken by the Executive

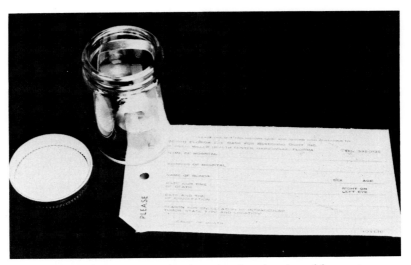

Figure 17-1. An eye bank moist chamber jar with an attached donor information card.

Director, who will coordinate eye collection and transportation. The eye bank will accept and obtain any eyes donated, regardless of cause of death, time postmortem, or donor age. Eyes not suitable for penetrating keratoplasty are used for lamellar grafts or for research.

DISTRIBUTION

Eyes collected by the eye bank are registered and processed for storage, preservation, or immediate shipping. Labels containing all adequate clinical information are affixed to the moist chamber jars (Fig. 17-1) or to vials with the cornea in M-K media. These are placed in the styrofoam shipping containers and packed with ice. Properly packed containers can maintain the +4°C temperature for over 24 hr.

Transportation of tissue secured from participating affiliated hospitals and funeral homes is provided by the Highway Patrol in many states. For example, Florida highway patrolmen will transport the styrofoam shipping containers from the pick-up point to the Emergency Room of the University of Florida Medical Center, and the eye bank is notified of their arrival.

REFERENCES

1. Dhanda RP, Kalevar V: Eye bank, In Dhanda RP, Kalevar V(eds): Corneal Surgery. International Ophthalmology Clinics. Boston, Little, Brown 1972
2. Sadler AM, Sadler BL: Transplantation and the Law: The need for organized sensitivity. Georgetown Law J 57:5, 1968

Bylaws of
North Florida Eye Bank for
Restoring Sight, Inc.

Directors

1.   The affairs of the Corporation shall be managed by a board of directors (hereinafter called the "board") consisting of not less than five nor more than 25 persons. Any vacancy on the board shall be filled by the affirmative vote by ballot of a majority of the remaining members of the board.

2.   Regular meetings of the board shall be held in June of each year at such times and places as the board shall by resolution establish.

3.   Special meetings of the board may be called by the president or any vice-president, and shall be called upon the written request of four directors.

4.   At least 10 days' notice of the time, place, and purpose of every meeting shall be given to all directors; but notice of meeting need not be given to any director if waived by him in writing, whether before or after such meeting is held, or if he shall be present at the meeting.

5.   A majority of the directors then in office shall constitute a quorum at any board meeting. Any director may be removed from office be a vote of two-thirds of the entire board.

ARTICLE II

Officers

1.   The officers of the Corporation shall consist of a president, one or more vice-presidents, a secretary, a treasurer, and such honorary vice-presidents, such assistant secretaries, and such assistant treasurers as the board may from time to time elect or designate.

2.   The officers shall be elected by ballot at the June meeting of the board and shall hold office until the next June meeting or until the election of their respective successors.

3.   The officers shall have such powers and duties as generally pertain to their several offices and as the president or board shall from time to time prescribe.

4.   Any officer may be removed from office by a vote of two-thirds of the entire board.

5.   The board may appoint a bank or trust company as assistant treasurer to be the depository of the seal, funds, and securities of the Corporation and of documents relating to the property of the Corporation. Any such assistant treasurer shall have such powers and duties as may from time to time be entrusted to it by the board.

ARTICLE III

Council

1.   The council of the Corporation shall consist of not more than 100 persons. Members of the council shall be selected by the board and shall hold office at the pleasure of the board.

2.   The council shall serve in an advisory capacity only.

3.   No regular meetings of the council shall be held, but special meetings may be called by the board, or by the president, or any vice-president.

4.   At least 10 days' notice of the time, place, and purpose of every meeting shall be given to all members of the council; but notice of meeting need not be given to any council member if waived by him in writing, whether before or after such meeting is held, or if he shall be present at the meeting.

ARTICLE IV

Committees

1.   The board may designate from its number an executive committee consisting of not less than three nor more than seven directors, which shall have and may exercise, when the board is not in session, all the powers of the board as far as permitted by law.

2.   The board may from time to time in its discretion appoint such other standing committees or temporary committees for such purposes as it may seem proper.

ARTICLE V

Members

1.   Members of the Corporation may be individuals, partnerships, or other corporations.

2.   There shall be the following classes of members: hospital members, annual members, contributing members, sustaining members, benefactor members, scholarship members, and fellowship members.

3.   Nominations for membership may be made by any director or any

member of the Corporation. Election to membership shall be subject to such rules as may from time to time be determined by the board.

4.   Any hospital corporation interested in the work of the Corporation shall be eligible for election as a hospital member.

5.   Any contributor to the work of the Corporation shall be eligible for election to the other classes of membership. Persons contributing from $2.00 to $10.00 in any one year shall be eligible for election as annual members for that year; persons contributing more than $10 and up to $25 in any one year shall be eligible for election as contributing members for that year; persons contributing more than $25 and up to $100 in any one year shall be eligible for election as sustaining members for that year; persons contributing more than $100 and up to $750 in any one year shall be eligible for election as benefactor members for that year; persons contributing more than $750 and up to $3,500 in any one year shall be eligible for election as scholarship members for that year; persons contributing more than $3,500 in any one year shall be eligible for election as fellowship members for that year.

6.   Any member may be expelled from membership by a vote of two-thirds of the entire board.

7.   Any member may resign from membership in the Corporation by written notice to its secretary.

ARTICLE VI

Liability of Members, Officers, and Directors

No member (of any class), officer, director, or member of the council of the Corporation, as such, shall be liable to the Corporation for any dues or subscription other than such as he may specifically agree to in writing.

ARTICLE VII

Seal

The seal of the Corporation may be affixed by any elected officer.

ARTICLE VIII

Amendments

These bylaws may be amended by a vote of two-thirds of the entire board at any meeting of the board, provided that notice of such amendment has been given at a previous meeting of the board and a copy of the proposed amendment sent to each director at least 10 days previous to the meeting at which the amendment is considered.

Amendments to Bylaws of North Florida Eye Bank for Restoring Sight, Inc.

Article I, Section 2 (providing for regular meeting) to read as follows:

ARTICLE I

2. Annual meetings of the board shall be held in the month of each year which and at such time as the Florida State Lions Convention is held. Other meetings of the board shall be held at such times and at such places as the board shall by resolution establish.

ARTICLE II, Section 2 (providing for election of officers) to read as follows:

ARTICLE II

2. The officers shall be elected by ballot at the annual meeting of the board and shall hold office until the next annual meeting or until the election of their respective successors.

I DO HEREBY CERTIFY that the above and foregoing are changes in the Bylaws of the North Florida Eye Bank for Restoring Sight, Inc., as adopted by a two-thirds vote of the members present at a regular Board of Directors meeting of the North Florida Eye Bank for Restoring Sight, Inc., at 2nd, Florida, March, 1974.

Amendment to Bylaws of North Florida Eye Bank for Restoring Sight, Inc.

Article VIII (method of amending bylaws) to read as follows:

ARTICLE VIII

Amendments

These bylaws may be amended by a vote of two-thirds of the members present at any meeting of the board, provided that notice of such amendment has been given at a previous meeting of the board and a copy of the proposed amendment sent to each director at least 10 days previous to the meeting at which the amendment is considered; and provided further that any such proposed amendment shall first be approved by a two-thirds vote of the Lions assembled at District meeting of Districts 35-F, 35-L, 35-0 and 35-R, Lions International, or by a two-thirds vote of the respective District cabinets of said Districts 35-F, 35-L, 35-0, and 35-R.

I DO HEREBY CERTIFY that the above and foregoing is a change in the bylaws of the North Florida Eye Bank for Restoring Sight, Inc., as adopted by a two-thirds vote of the members present at a regular Board of Directors meeting of the North Florida Eye Bank for Restoring Sight, Inc., at 3rd, Florida, March, 1974.

Amended Bylaws of the North Florida Lions Eye Bank for Restoring Sight, Inc.

ARTICLE I

Directors

1.   The affairs of the Corporation shall be managed by a board of directors (hereinafter called the "board") consisting of not less than five persons. Any vacancy on the board shall be filled by the Lions Club losing its member of the board and which created the vacancy, naming another one of its members to serve on the board, and said club shall notify the secretary of the corporation in writing of such action. A vacancy shall be deemed to have occurred if a member of the board of directors ceases to be a member of the Lions Club he represents. The filling of any such vacancy shall be for the balance of the unexpired term.

2.   Annual meetings of the board shall be held in the month of each year which and at such time as the Florida State Lions Convention is held. Other meetings of the board shall be held at such times and at such places as the board shall by resolution establish.

3.   Special meetings of the board may be called by the president or vice-president, and shall be called upon the written request of four directors.

4.   At least 10 days' notice of the time, place, and purpose of every meeting shall be given to all directors; but notice of meeting need not be given to any director if waived by him in writing, whether before or after such meeting is held, or if he shall be present at the meeting.

5.   A quorum at any meeting of the board of directors shall consist of those directors present. A majority of those directors present at any such meeting shall be required to pass on any matters coming before the board of directors.

6.   Any director may be removed from office at any regular or special meeting by vote of two-thirds of the directors present at such meeting.

7.   Any member of the board of directors who is absent from two successive meetings of the board, except with excused absence, shall be dropped as a director, his office declared vacant, and the Lions Club of Florida or Florida Lions Foundation for the Blind, Inc., as the case may be, shall replace said

member of the board, and notify the secretary of the Corporation in writing of such action. The filling of such vacancy shall be for the balance of the unexpired term.

8.   Any member of the board of directors who is unable to attend a regularly scheduled meeting may be represented by another member of his Club or Florida Lions Foundation for the Blind, Inc., as the case may be, upon presentation to the secretary of his authority to represent given by the president or secretary of his club or Florida Lions Foundation for the Blind, Inc., as the case may be, before attending such board meeting.

9.   There shall be an executive committee to act for the board of directors between regular board meetings, which executive committee shall consist of the president, vice-president, secretary, treasurer, immediate past president, and the district governors from subdistricts 35-F, 35-L, 35-0, Multiple District 35, Lions International, the current director representing the Florida Lions Foundation for the Blind, Inc., and the medical director of the Department of Ophthalmology, University of Florida, College of Medicine. Unless the board shall otherwise provide, the executive committee, during intervals between the meetings of the board of directors, may exercise powers of the full board of directors; and a majority of the members of the executive committee shall constitute a quorum for the transaction of such business as may come before the executive committee.

10.   The executive committee shall report to the board of directors at its regular meeting of any action taken by the executive committee between regular board meetings.

11.   The executive committee shall serve for a period of one year, or until their successors have been named.

12.   Any member of the executive committee may be removed from that office by a vote of two-thirds of the members in attendance at any executive committee meeting.

ARTICLE II

Officers

1.   The officers of the Corporation shall consist of a president, one or more vice-presidents, a secretary, a treasurer, and such honorary vice-presidents, such assistant secretaries, and such assistant treasurers as the board may from time to time elect or designate.

2.   The officers shall be elected by ballot at the annual meeting of the board and shall hold office until the next annual meeting or until the election of their respective successors.

3.   The officers shall have such powers and duties as generally pertain to their several offices and as the president or board shall from time to time prescribe.

4.   Any officer may be removed from office by a vote of two-thirds of the directors present at any regular meeting.

5.   The board may appoint a bank or trust company as assistant treasurer to

be the depository of the seal, funds, and securities of the Corporation and of documents relating to the property of the Corporation. Any such assistant treasurer shall have such powers and duties as may from time to time be entrusted to it by the board.

6. No compensation shall be paid to any officer or director of the Corporation, except that the board may employ an executive secretary and one or more technicians at such salary as may be determined by the board of directors. Travel expenses may be authorized by the board.

ARTICLE III

Council

1. The council of the Corporation shall consist of not more than 100 persons. Members of the council shall be selected by the board and shall hold office at the pleasure of the board.

2. The council shall serve in an advisory capacity only.

3. No regular meetings of the council shall be held, but special meetings may be called by the board or by the president, or any vice-president.

4. At least 10 days' notice of the time, place, and purpose of every meeting shall be given to all members of the council; but notice of meeting need not be given to any council member if waived by him in writing, whether before or after such meeting is held, or if he shall be present at the meeting.

ARTICLE IV

Committees

The president or the board may from time to time in its discretion appoint standing committees or temporary committees for such purposes as it may seem proper.

ARTICLE V

Members

1. Members of the Corporation shall be all Florida Lions in good standing, all members of the Department of Ophthalmology, University of Florida, College of Medicine, and any other interested individual, partnership, or corporation, as may be accepted by the board of directors.

2. Any member may be expelled from membership by a vote of two-thirds of the entire board.

3. Any member may resign from membership in the Corporation by written notice to its secretary.

ARTICLE VI

Liability of Members, Officers, and Directors

No member, officer, director, or member of the Corporation, as such, shall be liable to the Corporation for any dues or subscription other than such as he may specifically agree to in writing.

ARTICLE VII

Seal

The Corporation shall have a corporation seal.

ARTICLE VIII

Amendments

These bylaws may be amended by a vote of two-thirds of the directors present at any regular meeting of the board, provided that notice of such amendment has been given at a previous meeting of the board and a copy of the proposed amendment sent to each director at least 15 days previous to the meeting at which the amendment is to be considered.

ARTICLE IX

Fiscal Year and Limitations

1. The fiscal year of this Corporation shall commence July 1st each year.
2. This Corporation shall not participate in partisan or sectarian politics or religion.
3. The benefits of this Corporation shall be applied without discrimination for any reason to those within the scope of its activities.

ARTICLE IX

Membership

This corporation shall consist of not less than five members. Membership shall consist of all Florida Lions in good standing and members of the Department of Ophthalmology, University of Florida, College of Medicine. Any individual, partnership, or other corporation may become a member of this Corporation upon approval of a two-thirds vote of the Directors present at any regular meeting.

ARTICLE X

Amendments to the Articles of Incorporation

Any proposed amendments to the Articles of Incorporation may be made at any regular meeting of the board of directors upon a two-thirds vote of the directors present, provided that 15 days' notice shall have been given each individual member of the board of directors.

Index

Page numbers in *italics* refer to figures; page numbers followed by t refer to tables.